LMP

Last Minute Preparation

Obstetrics & Gynecology

for Postgraduates

LMP
Last Minute Preparation
Obstetrics & Gynecology
for Postgraduates

Editor

Mridu Sinha
MD (Obs and Gyne) MRCOG FACOG FMAS
Professor
Department of Obstetrics and Gynecology
Shri Ram Murti Smarak Institute of Medical Sciences
Bareilly, Uttar Pradesh, India

Co-Editors

Shashi Bala Arya
(Gold Medalist) MD (Obs and Gyne) FICOG
Professor and Head
Department of Obstetrics and Gynecology
Shri Ram Murti Smarak Institute of Medical Sciences
Bareilly, Uttar Pradesh, India

Namita Agarwal
MS (Obs and Gyne) FICOG FICMCH
Professor
Department of Obstetrics and Gynecology
Shri Ram Murti Smarak Institute of
Medical Sciences, Bareilly
Senior Consultant
Ekta Clinic
Bareilly, Uttar Pradesh, India

Manoj Kumar Tangri
MS (Obs and Gyne) Fellowship Gyne-Oncology
Professor
Department of Obstetrics and Gynecology
Shri Ram Murti Smarak Institute of
Medical Sciences
Bareilly, Uttar Pradesh, India

Forewords

Dev Murti, Mahendra Singh Butola, Shashi Bala Arya

JAYPEE

JAYPEE BROTHERS MEDICAL PUBLISHERS
The Health Sciences Publisher
New Delhi | London

Jaypee Brothers Medical Publishers (P) Ltd

Headquarters
Jaypee Brothers Medical Publishers (P) Ltd
EMCA House, 23/23-B
Ansari Road, Daryaganj
New Delhi 110 002, India
Landline: +91-11-23272143, +91-11-23272703
+91-11-23282021, +91-11-23245672
Email: jaypee@jaypeebrothers.com

Corporate Office
Jaypee Brothers Medical Publishers (P) Ltd
4838/24, Ansari Road, Daryaganj
New Delhi 110 002, India
Phone: +91-11-43574357
Fax: +91-11-43574314
Email: jaypee@jaypeebrothers.com

Overseas Office
JP Medical Ltd.
83, Victoria Street, London
SW1H 0HW (UK)
Phone: +44 20 3170 8910
Fax: +44 (0)20 3008 6180
Email: info@jpmedpub.com

Website: www.jaypeebrothers.com
Website: www.jaypeedigital.com

Inquiries for bulk sales may be solicited at: jaypee@jaypeebrothers.com

LMP Last Minute Preparation Obstetrics & Gynecology for Postgraduates

First Edition: **2025**

ISBN: 978-93-5696-843-1

Printed in India at Sterling Graphics Pvt. Ltd.

Contributors

Anuradha Sharma
DGO (KGMU) FMAS DMAS (Minimal Access Surgery) Fellowship in ART
Senior Consultant
Department of Obstetrics and Gynecology
Shri Ram Murti Smarak Institute of Medical Sciences
Bareilly, Uttar Pradesh, India

Babita Kumari
MS DNB (Obs and Gyne)
Assistant Professor
Department of Obstetrics and Gynecology
Shri Ram Murti Smarak Institute of Medical Sciences
Bareilly, Uttar Pradesh, India

Chanchal Choudhary
MS (Obs and Gyne)
Senior Resident
Department of Obstetrics and Gynecology
Shri Ram Murti Smarak Institute of Medical Sciences
Bareilly, Uttar Pradesh, India

Jyoti Baghel
MS (Obs and Gyne) DNB FMAS
Assistant Professor
Department of Obstetrics and Gynecology
Shri Ram Murti Smarak Institute of Medical Sciences
Bareilly, Uttar Pradesh, India

Manoj Kumar Tangri
MS (Obs and Gyne) Fellowship Gyne-Oncology
Professor
Department of Obstetrics and Gynecology
Shri Ram Murti Smarak Institute of Medical Sciences
Bareilly, Uttar Pradesh, India

Mridu Sinha
MD (Obs and Gyne) MRCOG FACOG FMAS
Professor
Department of Obstetrics and Gynecology
Shri Ram Murti Smarak Institute of Medical Sciences
Bareilly, Uttar Pradesh, India

Namita Agarwal
MS (Obs and Gyne) FICOG FICMCH
Professor
Department of Obstetrics and Gynecology
Shri Ram Murti Smarak Institute of Medical Sciences, Bareilly
Senior Consultant
Ekta Clinic
Bareilly, Uttar Pradesh, India

Parul Maheshwari
MS (Obs and Gyne)
Assistant Professor
Department of Obstetrics and Gynecology
Shri Ram Murti Smarak Institute of Medical Sciences
Bareilly, Uttar Pradesh, India

Pooja Mishra
MD (Obs and Gyne)
Assistant Professor
Department of Obstetrics and Gynecology
Shri Ram Murti Smarak Institute of Medical Sciences
Bareilly, Uttar Pradesh, India

Preeti Singh
MD (Obs and Gyne) PDCC (Maternal and Fetal Medicine)
Assistant Professor
Department of Obstetrics and Gynecology
Shri Ram Murti Smarak Institute of Medical Sciences
Bareilly, Uttar Pradesh, India

Ruchica Goel
DGO FICOG FICMCH DMAS FMAS
IVF Consultant
Department of Obstetrics and Gynecology
Shri Ram Murti Smarak Institute of Medical Sciences
Bareilly, Uttar Pradesh, India

Saumya Agarwal
MBBS MS (Obs and Gyne)
Senior Resident
Department of Obstetrics and Gynecology
Shri Ram Murti Smarak Institute of Medical Sciences
Bareilly, Uttar Pradesh, India

Shashi Bala Arya
(Gold Medalist) MD (Obs and Gyne) FICOG
Professor and Head
Department of Obstetrics and Gynecology
Shri Ram Murti Smarak Institute of Medical Sciences
Bareilly, Uttar Pradesh, India

Sunaina Chandra
MS (Obs and Gyne)
Senior Resident
Department of Obstetrics and Gynecology
Shri Ram Murti Smarak Institute of Medical Sciences
Bareilly, Uttar Pradesh, India

Surabhi Gupta
MS (Obs and Gyne)
Associate Professor
Department of Obstetrics and Gynecology
Shri Ram Murti Smarak Institute of Medical Sciences
Bareilly, Uttar Pradesh, India

Foreword

It is with great pleasure that, I introduce this invaluable resource, *LMP Last Minute Preparation Obstetrics & Gynecology for Postgraduates,* crafted by the dedicated professors of Shri Ram Murti Smarak Institute of Medical Sciences, Bareilly, Uttar Pradesh, India. As the Chairman of this esteemed institution, I have witnessed the unwavering commitment of our faculty to provide not just education, but also practical tools that enhance learning and clinical practice.

In the ever-evolving field of medicine, particularly in obstetrics and gynecology, staying updated with the latest knowledge and techniques is crucial. This book serves as an essential companion for postgraduate students, condensing vital information into an accessible format that can be utilized during the crucial moments of preparation. It encapsulates the expertise of our esteemed faculty, reflecting their collective experience and passion for teaching.

The structure of this book is designed to facilitate effective learning, enabling students to grasp complex concepts quickly and efficiently. It encourages not only memorization but also deeper understanding of the subjects that are fundamental to both the theory and practice of obstetrics and gynecology. This approach aligns the vision of fostering not only competent clinicians but also compassionate caregivers.

I encourage all postgraduate students to embrace this book as a guide during their studies. May it illuminate your path toward excellence in your medical career and inspire you to contribute to the well-being of women and families.

In conclusion, I extend my heartfelt congratulations to the authors for their efforts in compiling this work. It is my hope that this book will serve as a source of knowledge and confidence for many future healthcare professionals.

Warm regards,

Dev Murti
Chairman
Shri Ram Murti Smarak Institute of Medical Sciences
Bareilly, Uttar Pradesh, India

Foreword

I am glad the department of Obstetrics and Gynecology is publishing a book titled *"LMP Last Minute Preparation Obstetrics & Gynecology for Postgraduates."* I am sure this book will address the big issue of preparation for postgraduate (PG) examinations. As we all know, doing postgraduation in a subject like Obstetrics and Gynecology takes a big toll on the mental and physical faculty of the students because of the very busy schedule and long working hours. These postgraduates get very little time for preparation. Revising the subject before the examination is a challenging task.

I am confident that this book will be of great help to all the PG students preparing for their examination.

I compliment the entire team of authors to have thought of the requirement and worked hard to make it possible.

My best wishes for the success of the book.

Dr (Air Marshal) Mahendra Singh Butola (Retd.)
Principal
Shri Ram Murti Smarak Institute of Medical Sciences
Bareilly, Uttar Pradesh, India

Foreword

With great pleasure and responsibility, I feel honored to write the foreword for this handbook compiled for postgraduates by their compassionate teachers, keeping in mind their last-minute preparation. This book is not only a good tool to recall, remind, and revise by postgraduates but also helpful to the practicing clinicians. New recommendations and guidelines with references enhance the value of this book. Further, facilitation of content has been done with real-time photographs and inclusion of personal clinical experience wherever required.

Although this book cannot replace textbooks, I assure you that this handbook is a must-keep read in your reading shelf.

In the ever-evolving field of medicine, obstetrics and gynecology stands as a pillar of women's health, addressing the unique needs of half our population. This handbook encapsulates a pearl of knowledge on selected topics. The dedication and expertise of authors shine through in every chapter by addressing clinical protocols. I extend my deepest gratitude to the editor for her tireless efforts in bringing out this dream project.

May this handbook serve as a beacon of knowledge and testament to our unwavering commitment to women's health!

Shashi Bala Arya
Professor and Head
Department of Obstetrics and Gynecology
Shri Ram Murti Smarak Institute of Medical Sciences
Bareilly, Uttar Pradesh, India

Preface

It gives us an immense pleasure to bring forth our first handbook, designed especially for obstetrics and gynecology postgraduate (PG) junior residents! This book, which is in a short, concise, and crisp "notes" format, is being prepared by all teaching faculties of the Department of Obstetrics and Gynecology, Shri Ram Murti Smarak Institute of Medical Sciences, Bareilly, Uttar Pradesh, India. The context is being taken from various standard textbooks as well as the latest evidence-based recommendations from various guidelines like the Federation of Obstetric and Gynaecological Societies of India (FOGSI), the Royal College of Obstetricians and Gynaecologists (RCOG), the National Institute for Health and Care Excellence (NICE), the Faculty of Sexual and Reproductive Health (FSRH), the American College of Obstetricians and Gynecologists (ACOG), and the European Society of Human Reproduction and Embryology (ESHRE).

Being in the teaching profession, we always tried to make our subject "obstetrics and gynecology" interesting, captivating, and thought-provoking to whoever be our students—undergraduates or PG. Also, with respect to our PG residents working in obstetrics and gynecology, who are always on war front busy with their patients, they do not get enough time to go through different guidelines and their recommendations apart from their standard textbooks. This book will serve as a rapid revision tool, thereby making their last-minute preparation easy. So, with the idea that this will help them to keep abreast with the latest research and developments in a short-time span, we dedicate this book to them. We look forward to any suggestions or corrections, especially from PG residents, on how to make it better and thus help in achieving their milestones.

Mridu Sinha
Shashi Bala Arya
Namita Agarwal
Manoj Kumar Tangri

Acknowledgments

I, on behalf of my department—Obstetrics and Gynecology, Shri Ram Murti Smarak Institute of Medical Sciences, Bareilly, Uttar Pradesh, India, am grateful to all my teaching faculties, who have taken pain and extra effort despite their busy work and family life to contribute to this book. I am also grateful to my parents and brothers, who consistently supported me as pillars of strength. Last but not least, I am thankful to M/s Jaypee Brothers Medical Publishers (P) Ltd, New Delhi, India, who understood our very aim of bringing this book and published it in stipulated time.

Mridu Sinha

Contents

SECTION 12 SURGICAL SKILLS AND POSTOPERATIVE COMPLICATIONS

Section Authors: *Mridu Sinha, Jyoti Baghel, Chanchal Choudhary*

SECTION 1

Early Pregnancy

Section Authors: *Mridu Sinha, Pooja Mishra, Saumya Agarwal*

CHAPTER 1

Spontaneous Miscarriage/ Early Pregnancy Loss

DEFINITION

Nonviable intrauterine pregnancy, with either an empty gestational sac or a gestational sac (G. sac) containing an embryo without cardiac activity in the first 12–13 completed weeks of pregnancy. Incidence—10–15% of all clinically recognized pregnancies.

RISK FACTORS

- Advanced maternal age (>35 years), at age of 40 years it increases up to 50%
- Lifestyle factors such as obesity, smoking or heavy drinking
- Medical condition, e.g., uncontrolled diabetes, hypothyroidism
- History of previous miscarriage
- Fetal chromosomal anomalies. No evidence that stress or sex during pregnancy is causative.

INVESTIGATIONS

Transvaginal ultrasound (TVS) findings diagnostic of early pregnancy loss (EPL) are:

- Mean sac diameter (MSD) ≥25 mm with no embryo
- Crown-rump length (CRL) ≥7 mm with no cardiac activity
- Absence of embryo with heartbeat ≥11 days after scan showing G. sac with Yolk sac
- Absence of embryo with heartbeat ≥14 days after scan showing G. sac without Yolk sac.

According to the National Institute for Health and Care Excellence (NICE), if CRL is <7.0 mm on TVS and there is no visible heartbeat, perform a second scan a minimum of 7 days after the first; and if CRL ≥7.0 mm on TVS and there is no visible heartbeat, seek a second opinion on the viability of the pregnancy and/or perform a second scan a minimum of 7 days after the first before making a diagnosis.

If the mean gestational sac diameter (GSD) is <25.0 mm on TVS and there is no visible fetal pole, perform a second scan a minimum of 7 days after the first; and if the mean GSD ≥25.0 mm on TVS and there is no visible fetal pole, seek a second opinion on the viability of the pregnancy and/or perform a second scan a minimum of 7 days after the first for diagnosis.

MANAGEMENT

Expectant

Wait and watch for spontaneous expulsion till 7–14 days along with informed decision-making about the course (verbal and written), pain relief options, and to seek emergency help if there is increase in bleeding or pain or any signs of developing infection. Contraindications (CI)—if at increased risk of bleeding (e.g., in late first trimester or coagulopathies)/previous adverse and/or traumatic experience [e.g., stillbirth, miscarriage, or antepartum hemorrhage (APH)]/evidence of infection. If subsidence of bleeding and pain indicates miscarriage is completed during 7–14 days of expectant management, advise a urine pregnancy test at home, 3 weeks after their miscarriage, and to return for if it is positive. Repeat TVS if bleeding and/or pain not started or excessive and continuing suggestive of incomplete miscarriage. Success rate ~50%.

Medical

If patient not willing for expectant, no pain or bleeding or infection or anemia/coagulopathy, then 200 mg oral Mifepristone followed by 48 hours later (American College of Obstetricians and Gynecologists ACOG—24 hours), 800 µg Misoprostol (vaginal, oral, or sublingual) with analgesics and antiemetics SOS. Side-effects—pain, cramps, diarrhea, and vomiting. Advise to return back if excessive pain and/or bleeding per vaginum (PV), and also if bleeding does not start 48 hours after Misoprostol. Urine pregnancy test (UPT) after 3 weeks, and report back if positive to rule out retained product of conception, ectopic, or molar, also heavy bleeding, pain, or fever even if UPT is negative. Success rate ~85%.

Surgical

If patient is bleeding, hemodynamically unstable, having infection, medical disorders such as anemia, cardiovascular disease, and coagulopathies, or not responding to medical/expectant treatment. Manual vacuum aspiration (MVA) under local anesthesia/suction evacuation after verbal and written consent. Complications are injury to cervix/uterus (perforation), excessive bleeding, infection and rarely intrauterine adhesions due to excessive curettage. Prophylactic preoperative single dose of Doxycycline 100 mg 1 hour before is recommended to prevent infection. CI or intolerance to expectant and medical management is also the indication of surgical management, e.g., excessive/prolonged pain or bleeding, fever/sepsis. Success rate ~95%.

Role of Anti-D in Rh-ve pregnancy—recommended in surgical method [50 µg intramuscular (IM) in first trimester]. According to NICE, no Anti-D in threatened/complete miscarriage or those medically managed or pregnancy of unknown location; indicated only when surgically managed or associated with severe pain/bleeding.

Recurrence: No increased risk if only one/two miscarriages, but after three consecutive loss it increases to 40%.

Contraception: If patient desirous then both hormonal and intrauterine contraceptive device (CI—sepsis) can be advised just after completion of the process.

SUGGESTED READING

1. American College of Obstetricians and Gynecologists' Committee on Practice Bulletins—Gynecology. ACOG Practice Bulletin No. 200: Early Pregnancy Loss. Obstet Gynecol. 2018;132(5):e197-e207.
2. NICE guideline No. 126. Ectopic pregnancy and miscarriage: diagnosis and initial management. London: National Institute for Health and Care Excellence (NICE); 2023.

CHAPTER 2

Recurrent Miscarriage/ Recurrent Pregnancy Loss

DEFINITION

Spontaneous loss of ≥3 consecutive first trimester (or ≥1 second trimester) pregnancies <24 weeks. *Incidence:* 1%. Recurrent pregnancy loss (RPL) can be primary (never carried pregnancy to period of viability, i.e., 24 weeks or beyond) or secondary (women with previous live birth).

RISK FACTORS

- Age—both maternal (>35 years) and paternal (>40 years) (∵ decrease quality-quantity of gametes)
- Body mass index (BMI)—obesity (>30 kg/m^2)
- Lifestyle—alcohol (≥5 units/week) and smoking (caffeine-insufficient evidence)
- Occupation—conflicting evidence with use of anesthetic gases.
- Obstetric history—↑risk after each successive pregnancy loss (40% >3 consecutive pregnancy losses)
- Past medical history—uncontrolled thyroid/diabetes, thrombophilia (congenital/acquired).

CAUSES

- *Endocrine*—uncontrolled diabetes, thyroid dysfunction, polycystic ovary syndrome (PCOS) (possibly increased risk is attributed to insulin resistance, hyperinsulinemia, and hyperandrogenemia. Elevated free androgen index—prognostic factor for subsequent miscarriage).
- *Genetic*—Embryonic chromosomal abnormalities (30–57%), parental structural chromosomal anomaly (2–5%) (balanced reciprocal/Robertsonian translocation)
- *Antiphospholipid syndrome* (15% RPL)—interference with function and differentiation of trophoblasts, activation of complement pathways at maternal-fetal interface → local inflammation and thrombosis of uteroplacental vasculature.
- *Inherited thrombophilia*—Activated protein C resistance (factor V Leiden mutation), deficiencies of protein C/S and antithrombin III, hyperhomocysteinemia, and prothrombin gene mutation.
- *Anatomical*—Congenital uterine malformation, cervical incompetence.
- *Infection*—Bacterial vaginosis (BV) in first trimester is risk factor for second trimester miscarriage and preterm labor, but no evidence on TORCH (*Toxoplasma gondii*, Rubella, Cytomegalovirus, and Herpes simplex virus) infection for RPL, and bacteremia and viremia risk factor for sporadic miscarriage.
- *Immune causes*—No evidence on Human Leukocyte Antigens (HLA) incompatibility between couples, Natural Killer (NK) cells in peripheral blood or uterine.
- *Male factor*—Recent evidence shows that increased sperm Deoxyribonucleic acid (DNA) fragmentation may be a risk for miscarriage, but its role in RPL is unclear [American Society for Reproductive Medicine (ASRM)].

APPROACH

- *History taking regarding previous losses*—Gestational age, fetal cardiac activity in ultrasonography (USG), painful/painless in second trimester loss.
- *Physical examination*—Signs of endocrinopathy—hirsutism, galactorrhea; pelvic examination to rule out uterine malformation, cervical laceration, etc.
- *Investigations:*
    - Serum thyroid-stimulating hormone (TSH), fasting blood sugar (FBS)/post-prandial blood sugar (PPBS)
    - Antiphospholipid Antibody Syndrome (APLAS)—Sapporo criteria—Antiphospholipid Antibodies (APA) + any adverse pregnancy outcome/vascular thrombosis.
        - APA—Lupus Anticoagulant (LAC), Anticardiolipin Antibodies (ACA), and Anti-B2 glycoprotein-I antibodies (present on 2 occasions 12 weeks apart).
        - Adverse pregnancy outcomes—≥3 consecutive miscarriages <10 weeks of gestation/≥1

morphologically normal fetal loss >10 weeks/ ≥1 preterm birth (PTB) <34 weeks owing to placental disease.
- Combined hysterolaparoscopy/3D USG—congenital uterine malformation
- Free androgen index in PCOS (prognostic factor)
- Product of conception in third miscarriage for embryonic chromosomal abnormalities, and if positive then parental karyotyping (Balanced translocation).

MANAGEMENT

Recurrent miscarriage clinic. Lifestyle modification such as reducing BMI in obese, avoidance of tobacco products, alcohol, and excess caffeine.

- *APLAS*—Low-dose Aspirin (LDA) + Heparin [low-molecular-weight Heparin (LMWH)] once pregnancy test is positive till 34 weeks. Side-effects of Heparin—bleeding, hypersensitivity reactions, thrombocytopenia, osteopenia, and vertebral fractures on long-term use [live birth rates (LBRs) improves].
- *Genetic cause*—Refer to genetic counselor
  - Options
    - Natural pregnancy with/without prenatal diagnostic tests (amniocentesis/chorionic villus sampling (CVS)]
    - In vitro fertilization (IVF) with preimplantation genetic diagnosis (PGD)
    - Gamete (egg/sperm) or embryo donation or surrogacy
  - Adoption [50–70% chance of a healthy live birth in future natural pregnancies than after PGD (~30%)]
- *Inherited thrombophilia*—Insufficient role of Heparin in first trimester miscarriages, but may improve LBR in second trimester miscarriages with inherited thrombophilia.
- *Immunotherapy*—No role except for research purposes [paternal cell immunization, donor leukocytes, trophoblast membranes, intravenous (IV) immunoglobulin] (Grade 1A).
- *Endocrine factors*—Diabetic control and thyroid dysfunction correction decreases miscarriage, but insufficient evidence on progesterone, human Chorionic Gonadotropin (hCG), Metformin, suppression of Luteinizing Hormone (LH) hypersecretion, or correction of hyperprolactinemia. Vaginal Micronized progesterone 400 mg BD has modest benefit in those presenting with early bleeding (i.e., threatened miscarriage) along with history of RPL (Grade 2B).
- *Bacterial vaginosis infection*—Screening and treatment of infection in first trimester of women with history of second trimester loss and/or preterm labor may reduce late miscarriages and preterm labor.
- *Cervical incompetence*—History indicated cerclage in those with singleton pregnancy and history of ≥3 second trimester loss. USG-indicated cerclage, if cervical length of ≤25 mm detected by transvaginal ultrasound (TVS) before 24 weeks of gestation in women with singleton pregnancy and history of one mid-trimester miscarriage.
- *Uterine abnormalities*—Surgical correction of uterine septum, intrauterine adhesions, or submucous leiomyoma (hysteroscopically).
- *Unexplained RPL*—with supportive tender loving care 75% achieve a successful future pregnancy.

NOT RECOMMENDED

- *Investigations*—TORCH test, routine parental karyotyping, HLA, blood NK cells, cytokines, cervical weakness test. No routine thyroid function test (TFT)/ thyroid antibodies test or screening for diabetes in asymptomatic women.
- *Treatment*—Corticosteroids (Grade 1B), IV immunoglobulins, hCG, Metformin, progesterone, pre-pregnancy suppression of high LH levels among ovulatory women with RPL and polycystic ovaries, Heparin to prevent first trimester miscarriage associated with inherited thrombophilia, and Aspirin alone or in combination with Heparin for unexplained RPL.

SUGGESTED READING

1. Chester MR, Tirlapur A, Jayaprakasan K. Current management of recurrent pregnancy loss. Obstet Gynaecol. 2022;24: 260-71.
2. Dhillon-Smith RK, Boelaert K, Jeve YB, Maheshwari A, Coomarasamy A; Royal College of Obstetricians and Gynaecologists. Subclinical hypothyroidism and antithyroid autoantibodies in women with subfertility or recurrent pregnancy loss. Scientific Impact Paper No. 78. BJOG. 2022;129:e75-e88.
3. Regan L, Rai R, Saravelos S, Li T-C; Royal College of Obstetricians and Gynaecologists. Recurrent Miscarriage Green - top guideline No. 17. BJOG. 2023; 130(12):e9-e39.

CHAPTER 3

Molar Pregnancy

GESTATIONAL TROPHOBLASTIC DISEASE

A condition characterized by abnormal trophoblast proliferation which produces excess amount of pregnancy hormone—human chorionic gonadotropin (hCG)—crucial for gestational trophoblastic disease (GTD) diagnosis, management, and surveillance.

MODIFIED WORLD HEALTH ORGANIZATION CLASSIFICATION OF GESTATIONAL TROPHOBLASTIC DISEASES

Molar Pregnancies—Hydatidiform Mole

- Complete mole
- Partial mole
- Invasive mole

Table 1 shows the main differences between complete mole and partial mole.

TABLE 1: Difference between partial and complete molar pregnancy.

Feature	*Partial mole*	*Complete mole*
Karyotype	69,XXX or 69,XXY	46,XX
Clinical presentation:		
Diagnosis	Missed abortion	Molar gestation
Uterine size	Small for date	Large for date
Theca lutein cyst	Rare	25–30% of cases
Initial hCG level	<100,000 mIU/mL	>100,000 mIU/mL
Medical complication	Rare	Uncommon
Rate of subsequent GTN	1–5% of cases	15–20% of cases
Pathology:		
Embryo-fetus	Often present	Absent
Amnion-fetal erythrocyte	Often present	Absent
Villous edema	Focal	Widespread
Trophoblastic proliferation	Focal, slight-to-moderate	Slight to severe
Trophoblast atypia	Mild	Marked
P57KIP2 immunostaining	Positive	Negative

(GTN: gestational trophoblastic neoplasia; hCG: human chorionic gonadotropin)

Trophoblastic Tumor

- Choriocarcinoma
- Placental site trophoblastic tumor
- Epithelioid trophoblastic tumor

MEDICAL COMPLICATIONS

Anemia, hyperthyroidism, hyperemesis gravidarum, preeclampsia, and infection.

RISK FACTORS

The strongest risk factors are age—both at extremes of reproductive life, and history of prior hydatidiform mole.

CLINICAL FINDINGS

History

- Amenorrhea
- Bleeding per vaginal (may lead to profuse hemorrhage)
- Nausea and vomiting, or hyperemesis
- Features of hyperthyroidism, early-onset preeclampsia and abdominal distension due to theca lutein cysts.
- Rarely with hemoptysis/seizures due to involvement of lungs or brain.

Physical Findings

- Uterine growth more than gestational age
- Soft in consistency
- No fetal movement with complete moles.
- Serum free thyroxine (fT4) ↑ and thyroid-stimulating hormone (TSH) ↓
- Severe preeclampsia and eclampsia are relatively common with advanced molar pregnancies.

Sonography

A complete mole appears as an echogenic uterine mass filling the endometrial cavity with no fetus or gestational sac, composed of numerous anechoic cystic spaces of different sizes and shapes. This appearance is often described as a *"snowstorm."*

A partial mole has features that include a thick, multicystic placenta plus a fetus, or fetal tissue. Definitive diagnosis by histopathological examination. Ultrasonography (USG) shows cystic spaces in the placenta, and ratio of transverse to antero-posterior dimension of the gestational sac greater than 1:1.5.

MANAGEMENT

Investigation

- Hemogram
- Beta-hCG
- Serum TSH, free thyroxine (FT4)
- Blood grouping
- Chest X-ray
- Ultrasonography pelvis

TREATMENT

Irrespective of gestational age/uterine size, uterine evacuation by *suction curettage* is the preferred treatment, better under USG guidance to decrease the risk of uterine perforation. Role of Oxytocin infusion during surgical removal—routine preoperative use is not recommended but should be used only when significant bleeding prior to or during removal, to decrease risk of tissue embolization.

Anti-D immunoglobulin (RhoGAM) to Rh D negative women.

POSTEVACUATION SURVEILLANCE

Due to risk for subsequent gestational trophoblastic neoplasia (GTN) following molar pregnancy, postevacuation surveillance is indicated. Serial measurement of serum β-hCG levels aim to detect persistent or renewed trophoblastic proliferation.

- *The initial serum β-hCG level:* Within 48 hours of evacuation.
- There after every 1–2 weeks. Levels are followed until they become undetectable, usually 56 days, then monthly determinations for 6 months. If β-hCG does not normalize within 56 days, then 6-month follow-up done from date of normalization.
- For partial mole follow-up concluded once it is normal on two occasions 4 weeks apart.

Women are advised not to conceive till their follow-up is complete, i.e., 6 months after normalization of β-hCG, when monitoring is discontinued and pregnancy allowed. During follow-up reliable *contraception* is advised to avoid confusion caused by rising β-hCG levels from a new pregnancy. Hormonal contraception either in form of combined oral contraceptive (COC) pills, injection Depot Medroxyprogesterone Acetate (DMPA) or progestin implant can be given. Intrauterine devices are not used until β-hCG levels are undetectable because of the risk of uterine perforation.

SUGGESTED READING

1. Berek JS. Berek & Novak's Gynecology, 17th edition. Philadelphia: Wolters Kluwer; 2022.
2. Tidy J, Seckl M, Hancock BW. Management of gestational trophoblastic disease. BJOG. 2021;128:e1-e27.

CHAPTER 4

Hyperemesis Gravidarum

NAUSEA AND VOMITING OF PREGNANCY

This is defined as the symptom of nausea and/or vomiting during pregnancy, beginning before 16 weeks of gestation after exclusion of other causes. *Incidence*—90% pregnancies. In majority of women (90%), it starts between 4th and 7th weeks of gestation, peaks in 9th week and resolves by the 20th week of pregnancy.

HYPEREMESIS GRAVIDARUM

Severe form of nausea and vomiting of pregnancy (NVP), affects the quality of life by interfering with eating and drinking normally, thus limiting daily living activities with or without signs of dehydration. *Incidence*—0.3–3%.

PATHOLOGY

Both NVP and hyperemesis gravidarum (HG) occurs due to increased sensitivity to vomiting hormone—growth differentiation factor-15 (GDF-15) causing loss of appetite, altered taste, nausea, vomiting, and weight loss. Genetic variants of GDF-15 [not human chorionic gonadotropin (hCG)] are associated with increased risk for HG and also associated with recurrence in next pregnancies. Both are associated with $\downarrow Na^+$, $\downarrow K^+$, ↓urea, ↑Hct, and ketonuria with metabolic hypochloremic alkalosis initially, may develop metabolic acidosis later.

APPROACH

History Taking

Previous obstetric history of NVP/HG, quantify severity using *Pregnancy-Unique Quantification of Emesis and Nausea (PUQE)-24 scoring* [*in last 24 hours—number of times vomiting and/or retching, times feeling nauseated—mild (6), moderate (7-12), and severe (13-15)*] or *HyperEmesis Level Prediction tool* [*HELP score—mild (≤19), moderate (20-32), and severe (33-60)*] which also helps to determine treatment response: nausea, vomiting, ptyalism (hypersalivation), spitting, weight loss, unable to tolerate food and fluids, affecting quality of life and daily activities, and nutritional status. Comorbidities are further complicated by lack of oral intake of essential medications such as diabetes, epilepsy, human immunodeficiency virus (HIV), psychiatric or mental conditions, and hypoadrenalism. Surgical history such as gastric bypass, band, or sleeve gastrectomy. Rule out other causes of abdominal pain, urine infection, and proper drug history (prescription and/or recreational).

On Examination

Pulse (tachycardia in dehydration), blood pressure (hypotension in dehydration), temperature, respiratory rate (RR) (tachypnea in dehydration), oxygen saturation (SpO_2), and weight. Rule out signs of malnutrition/dehydration—(sunken eyes, dry lips and mouth, oliguria, or anuria) or history of rapid weight loss (≥5% prepregnancy weight). Look for muscle wasting by measuring mid-arm circumference. Also see the neurological signs of Wernicke's encephalopathy (confusion, nystagmus, and ataxia).

INVESTIGATION

- Urinalysis—nitrites indicate infection (presence or absence of ketonuria in pregnancy is not an indicator of dehydration) and mid-stream urine (MSU) [if dipstick indicates signs of urinary tract infection (UTI)].
- Blood urea and serum electrolytes—to guide intravenous (IV) fluid and electrolyte replacement.
- Full blood count to rule out infection, anemia, and hematocrit.
- Plasma glucose level to rule out diabetes and diabetic ketoacidosis.
- Ultrasonography (USG) obstetric for viability of intrauterine pregnancy and/or rule out multiple pregnancy or trophoblastic disease.
- In refractory cases or history of recurrence, check thyroid function tests—hypothyroid/hyperthyroid.
- Liver function tests (LFTs) for hepatitis or gallstones.
- Calcium and phosphate level in blood.

- Serum amylase to exclude pancreatitis.
- Arterial blood gas (ABG) to exclude severe metabolic disturbances.

MANAGEMENT

Mild NVP who are not dehydrated are cared in community/ primary care with antiemetics, reassurance, oral hydration, and dietary advice (eat small, frequent meals to prevent an empty stomach). If unable to take oral fluids/ oral antiemetics then ambulatory day care management is done with IV fluids, vitamins (especially B1-thiamine) and parenteral antiemetics. Inpatient care done if continued nausea and vomiting and unable to take anything orally, associated with clinical dehydration or significant weight loss (>5% of body weight), despite oral antiemetics, confirmed or suspected any comorbidity—such as UTI and unable to tolerate oral antibiotics, diabetes, epilepsy, human immunodeficiency virus (HIV), hypoadrenalism, or psychiatric disease.

PHARMACOTHERAPY

Various medications have different mechanisms of action and so they work synergistically if combination antiemetics are used in women who do not respond to a single agent, from first-and second-line options.

- First-line drugs—Doxylamine and Pyridoxine, Cyclizine, Prochlorperazine, Promethazine, and Chlorpromazine.
- Second-line—Metoclopramide, Domperidone, and Ondansetron.
- Third-line—Hydrocortisone IV followed by oral Prednisolone.
- Corticosteroids are reserved for severe cases where first-and second-line medications are not effective and used along with antiemetics.
- H2 receptor blockers or proton pump inhibitors (PPI) used for gastroesophageal reflux disease (GERD), esophagitis, or gastritis.
- Thiamine (vitamin B_1)—oral 100 mg TDS or IV (part of vitamin B complex) should be given to decrease Wernicke encephalopathy (blurred vision, unsteadiness, confusion/memory problems/drowsiness, nystagmus, ophthalmoplegia, hyporeflexia/ areflexia, gait disturbances, and/or finger–nose ataxia).
- Low-molecular-weight Heparin (LMWH) for thromboprophylaxis, laxatives for constipation but avoid iron preparation. Normal saline (0.9% NaCl) with additional Potassium Chloride (KCl) guided by daily monitoring of electrolytes, is the most appropriate IV hydration, but avoid Dextrose infusion.

SIDE-EFFECTS

No risk of congenital malformations or other adverse pregnancy outcomes with first-line drugs, but a very small risk of orofacial clefting with Ondansetron use in first trimester. Extrapyramidal symptoms and oculogyric crises may occur with Phenothiazines and Metoclopramide. To decrease risk of dystonic reactions, injection Metoclopramide should only be used for short-term [*maximum dose of 30 mg in 24 hours or 0.5 mg/kg body weight in 24 hours (whichever is lowest) and for 5 days*] and it should be given by slow bolus injection over at least 3 minutes.

Postnatal depression (PND), anxiety, and post-traumatic stress disorder (PTSD) associated with severity of HG. When all medical therapies failed, enteral tube feeding, or parenteral treatment should be considered with referral to gastroenterology and multidisciplinary team (MDT). Medical termination of pregnancy (MTP) should be considered after all therapeutic measures have been offered.

Next pregnancy—*recurrence risk (15–81%)* hence, early use of lifestyle or dietary modifications and antiemetics.

SUGGESTED READING

1. RCOG Green-top Guideline No. 69. Management of nausea and vomiting in pregnancy and hyperemesis gravidarum. [online] Available from https://www.rcog.org.uk/guidance/browse-all-guidance/green-top-guidelines/the-management-of-nausea-and-vomiting-of-pregnancy-and-hyperemesis-gravidarum-green-top-guideline-no-69/ [Last accessed September, 2024].

CHAPTER 5

MTP Act, Amendment 2021

INTRODUCTION

Approximately 8% of maternal mortality is due to unsafe abortion. Hence, National Health Policy is to make abortion safe and widely available. The Medical Termination of Pregnancy (MTP) Act, enacted in India 1971, governs the provision of abortions in India.

DEVELOPMENT PROCESS

- *MTP Act 1971, amended 2002*—Passed by both houses of parliament and received assent by the President. Salient features are—indications of MTP, who and where can be done.
- *MTP rules 1975, amended 2003*—Made by central government and passed by parliament, notified in official gazette. Salient features—*District level committee:* composition and site approval, equipment required at sites, and experience and training required by registered medical practitioner (RMP).
- *MTP regulations 1975, amended 2003*—Made by state government and passed by state legislature. Salient features—Documentation and reporting.

WHEN PREGNANCY CAN BE TERMINATED

Neither abortion (MTP service) is available on demand nor it is a woman's right, also not done for sex selection, it should be done only for following indications, if:

- Continuation of pregnancy is a risk to the life of the pregnant woman or can cause grave injury to her physical or mental health, e.g., contraceptive failure (unmarried also), rape victims, or incest.
- Substantial risk that the child, if born, would be seriously handicapped due to physical or mental abnormalities.
- Women with major physical disabilities as laid under "Rights of persons with Disability Act, 2016."
- Minors
- Change in marital status during ongoing pregnancy (widow/divorce).
- Humanitarian grounds such as pregnancy during emergency/pandemic.
- Mentally ill women including mental retardation.

A pregnancy can be terminated at any period of gestation, if considered by the Medical Board on substantial fetal abnormalities. Medical Board consists of—1 gynecologist, 1 pediatrician, 1 radiologist/sonologist, and other members notified in Official Gazette by State Government/Union Territories Time frame—Medical Board decides in 3 days and MTP done in 5 days. In other cases, >24 weeks by written petition to court of law.

EXPERIENCE TO TERMINATE PREGNANCY

Only an RMP, possessing a recognized medical qualification and his/her name entered in State/National Medical Council can perform with following experience:

- Postgraduate degree/diploma in obstetrics and gynecology (Obs & Gyne).
- Completed 6 months as House Surgeon in Obs & Gyne.
- At least 1 year experience in the practice of Obs & Gyne at any hospital that has all facilities.
- One who has assisted an RMP in 25 cases of MTP of which at least five have been performed independently in a hospital established or maintained by the government or a training institute approved for this purpose (first trimester only).

CONSENT FOR MEDICAL TERMINATION OF PREGNANCY

Taken only on *Form C* with following conditions fulfilled:

- In case of a woman >18 years, married/unmarried, only the consent of the woman is required to terminate pregnancy.
- In case of a minor (<18 years) or a mentally-ill person, consent of a guardian is required.
  Spousal consent is not mandatory.

TABLE 1: Differences between MTP Act, 1971 and MTP Amendment, 2021.

	The MTP Act 1971	*The MTP Amendment Act 2021*
Indications (contraceptive failure)	Only applies to married women	Unmarried women are also covered
Gestational age limit	20 weeks for all indications	24 weeks for rape survivors; beyond 24 weeks for substantial fetal abnormalities
Medical practitioner opinions required before termination	• One RMP till 12 weeks • Two RMPs till 20 weeks	• One RMP till 20 weeks • Two RMPs 20–24 weeks • Medical board approval after 24 weeks
Breach of the woman's confidentiality	Fine up to INR 1,000	Fine and/or imprisonment of 1 year

(MTP: Medical Termination of Pregnancy; RMP: registered medical practitioner)

GESTATIONAL AGE TO TERMINATE PREGNANCY

- For termination of pregnancy up to 12 weeks, opinion of 1 RMP is required.
- For termination of pregnancy between 13 and 20 weeks, opinions of 2 RMPs are required.
- *According to amendment 2021*, up to 20 weeks—1 RMP opinion; between 20 and 24 weeks, opinions of 2 RMP are required; and >24 weeks state-level Medical Board will decide.

SITE FOR PREGNANCY TERMINATION

Any government hospital or private clinic approved by the government/district level committee. As per national guidelines, pregnancy can be terminated at government centers as up to—8 weeks at primary health center (PHC), 12 weeks at community health center (CHC), and 20 weeks at district hospital and above.

MANDATORY DOCUMENTATION UNDER THE MEDICAL TERMINATION OF PREGNANCY ACT

- *Form "C":* Consent form
- *RMP opinion form:*
  - Form I—up to 20 weeks pregnancy termination (signed by 1 RMP)
  - Form E—for 20 to 24 weeks pregnancy termination (signed by 2 RMP)
  - Form D—beyond 24 weeks pregnancy termination, by Medical Board approval.
- *Form II:* Head of the hospital/owner of the place will send a monthly report of cases to the chief medical officer (CMO) of district.
- *Form III (Admission register):* Confidential document to maintain case records done at that site, no documentation in case-sheet, operation theater (OT) register, follow-up card, or any other register other than admission register. This register is kept for 5 years from the date of last entry.

These forms and documents are **not** used for other types of abortion, e.g., spontaneous, inevitable, incomplete, and missed abortion. Any violation of MTP act by person/place/documents is punishable with rigorous imprisonment for 2–7 years.

Table 1 shows the changes in Amendment Act, 2021 of MTP. According to the act—name and other particulars of a woman seeking MTP shall not be revealed except to a person authorized by law. Amendment act, 2021 benefits are—As many fetal abnormalities are detected >20 week scan, it will cater such cases; allows rape victims, minors and disabled women to abort unwanted pregnancies safely and legally; also allows unmarried woman to legally terminate without disclosing their identity (term "*husband*" is replaced by "*partner*").

MTP in minor—must inform police as per POCSO Act, can do procedure with consent of adult guardian, rest same.

SUGGESTED READING

1. Gandhi A. Maheshwari B. FOGSI FOCUS on medical termination of pregnancy (MTP), Recent update on clinical and legal aspects; 2020.

CHAPTER 6

Pregnancy of Unknown Location

DEFINITION

Clinical entity in which there is no sign of either intrauterine or extrauterine pregnancy or retained product of conception on transvaginal ultrasound (TVS), despite positive pregnancy test. It requires continued evaluation till a final diagnosis is reached, i.e., live intrauterine pregnancy (IUP) or miscarriage or ectopic. Rarely when location never confirmed, will either have—(1) Spontaneously resolving/failing pregnancy of unknown location (PUL)—β-human chorionic gonadotropin (hCG) concentration normalizes without surgical or medical intervention, or (2) Persisting PUL—β-hCG concentration do not normalize with no evidence of trophoblastic disease/location of pregnancy by TVS (usually serum β-hCG <500 IU/L and reached plateau, doubling time >7 days).

FINAL OUTCOME

Final outcome could be:

- Intrauterine pregnancy (IUP—live/demise)
- Ectopic
- Failing PUL
- Persisting PUL
- Molar/trophoblastic disease
- Rarely—malignancy (invasive mole or choriocarcinoma)/pituitary or postcranial fossa tumor/heterophile antibodies/lab error.

CLINICAL PRESENTATION

- Asymptomatic, diagnosed incidentally during evaluation.
- Symptomatic—early pregnancy (nausea, vomiting, fatigue, and breast discomfort) or miscarriage (bleeding per vaginum) or ectopic (pain lower abdomen, irregular bleeding per vaginum).

EVALUATION

- *History taking:* Menstrual history for last menstrual period (LMP) and cycle-length, risk factors for ectopic [previous ectopic, tubal pathology, or surgery, intrauterine contraceptive device (IUCD), in vitro fertilization (IVF) conception, and smoking].
- *Examination:* General, per abdomen, pelvic examination to rule out adnexal mass suggestive of ectopic or miscarriage (bleeding from cervical os).

INVESTIGATION

Serum β-hCG on D-0 and repeat after 48 hours, TVS—if β-hCG above discriminatory zone (or symptomatic) with no intrauterine gestational sac to rule out ectopic (extrauterine gestational sac or complex adnexal mass or echogenic fluid), complete blood count (CBC) (if bleeding), renal function test (RFT), and (liver function test) LFT (if required treatment with Methotrexate), Rh typing (for Anti-D).

MANAGEMENT

If patient is hemodynamically stable and asymptomatic → conservative treatment with serial serum β-hCG every 48 hours. If level of β-hCG rising >63% (or doubling) it is suggestive of early IUP, → Offer TVS scan to determine the location of the pregnancy between 7 and 14 days later. Consider an earlier scan for women with a serum hCG level ≥1,500 IU/L [National Institute for Health and Care Excellence (NICE)-2019, amended, 2023]. If visualized, no further β-hCG needed and repeat TVS 1–2 weeks after for fetal viability.

If level of β-hCG falling >50%, suggestive of failing PUL → ask her to take a urine pregnancy test 14 days after the second serum hCG test, and explain that—if the test is negative, no further action is necessary—if the test is positive, she should return to the early pregnancy assessment service for clinical review within 24 hours (NICE-2012) or repeat hCG >1 week to confirm failing PUL, then weekly till <10 IU/L, no further TVS required.

If serum β-hCG rising but <63% or falling <50% (suboptimal), then serial β-hCG till >1,000 IU/L or three measurements showing suboptimal ↑/↓ or plateauing/fluctuating or patient becomes symptomatic → repeat TVS to rule out ectopic → if still negative ultrasonography (USG), then it is managed as persisting PUL and needs Methotrexate 50 mg/m^2 intramuscular (IM) (especially if asymptomatic, with prior blood investigation done—CBC/LFT and RFT). 75% patient may feel pain abdomen on D3-7 (if excessive pain then rule out tubal rupture/ruptured ectopic), β-hCG may increase D1–4, mean time to resolution is 35 days. Single injection of Methotrexate is well tolerated, side-effects are minimal and pregnancy should be avoided for 3 months.

If the patient is hemodynamically unstable (e.g., ruptured ectopic or bleeding due to miscarriage) or becomes symptomatic anytime during conservative treatment or at time of presentation or if ectopic pregnancy is visualized on TVS, then immediate fluid resuscitation and surgical treatment is indicated—laparoscopy/laparotomy, and/or uterine evacuation.

SPECIAL CONSIDERATIONS

Patients with persistent β-hCG elevations or with nonpregnancy-related cause (e.g., pituitary production, heterophilic antibodies, etc.) are managed differently according to their final diagnosis.

SUGGESTED READING

1. National Institute for Health and Care Excellence: Guidelines. Ectopic pregnancy and miscarriage: diagnosis and initial management (NG126). London: National Institute for Health and Care Excellence (NICE); 2023.
2. Sagili H, Mohamed K. Pregnancy of unknown location: an evidence-based approach to management. Obstet Gynaecol. 2008;10:224-30.
3. Topic 134770 Version 5.0. https://www.uptodate.com/contents/approach-to-the-patient-with-pregnancy-of-unknown-location?search=Approach%20to%20the%20patient%20with%20pregnancy%20of%20unknown%20location&source=search_result&selected Title=1%7E150&usage_type=default&display_rank=1.

NOTES

NOTES

SECTION 2

Antenatal Care

Section Authors: *Namita Agarwal, Mridu Sinha, Surabhi Gupta, Chanchal Choudhary*

CHAPTER 7

Antepartum Fetal Surveillance

DEFINITION

Assessment of in utero fetal wellbeing prior to the onset of labor, to reduce perinatal morbidity and mortality. Timely detection and management prevent it, as the most common cause is uteroplacental insufficiency. Current testing protocols for high-risk pregnancies attempt to distinguish fetuses that can be safely managed expectantly from those which need to be delivered promptly.

Current testing options are:

- The fetal movement counts
- Nonstress test (NST)
- Cardiotocography (CTG)
- Vibroacoustic stimulation test
- Contraction stress test
- Nipple stimulation test
- Biophysical profile (BPP)
- Doppler study
- Fetal lung maturation test

LIMITATIONS

Acute cord accidents, maternal trauma, accidental hemorrhage and rupture of the uterus cannot be predicted in advance by these tests. In addition, congenital anomalies, which contribute significantly to perinatal and neonatal mortality rates, cannot be entirely prevented.

TIME OF STARTING ANTENATAL SURVEILLANCE

It depends on past obstetric history and the severity of maternal and fetal condition. In majority of high-risk pregnancies, it is begun from 32 to 34 weeks onward. However, it can be started early at 26–28 weeks in more severe cases and repeated weekly or earlier depending on the risk. In normal pregnancy, it begins at 36 weeks.

INDICATIONS

- *Maternal conditions:* Antiphospholipid syndrome, poorly controlled hyperthyroidism, hemoglobinopathies such as hemoglobin SS, SC or S-thalassemia, cyanotic heart disease, systemic lupus erythematosus, chronic renal disease, diabetes mellitus, and hypertensive disorders.
- *Pregnancy-related conditions:* Gestational hypertension, preeclampsia, decreased fetal movement, oligohydramnios, polyhydramnios, intrauterine growth restriction (IUGR), post-term pregnancy, moderate-to-severe isoimmunization, previous fetal demise (unexplained or recurrent risk), and multiple gestation with significant growth discrepancy.
- *Fetal conditions:* IUGR, isoimmunization, and hydrops fetalis.

TECHNIQUES

Fetal Movement Counts by the Mother

Maternal perception of fetal movement is an inexpensive and noninvasive method of assessing fetal wellbeing. Studies have shown that fetal movement counts are an effective screening measure, with reported reductions in fetal mortality from 8.7 deaths/1,000 live births to 2 deaths/1,000 live births.

Methods of Assessment of Fetal Movement

- *Daily fetal movement count (DFMC):* Mother is asked to lie on left lateral side after eating—breakfast, lunch, and dinner, and to concentrate on fetal movements three times a day for 30–60 minutes. <3 fetal movements/hour on 2 consecutive days requires further evaluation [FM × 4 = DFMC/12 hours (Normal is 10 FM in 12 hours)]

- Cardiff count to 10—mother is asked to start counting fetal movements in the morning and record the time at which the tenth movement occurs. >10 movements/ 12 hours are normal.

Perception of fetal movement decreased in cases of obesity, anterior placenta, hydramnios, congenital abnormalities, maternal activity, and maternal medications, e.g., barbiturates and narcotics.

Nonstress Test

The principle of test is that the heart rate of the normal fetus (not acidotic/neurologically depressed) will temporarily accelerate with fetal movement. Loss of reactivity is commonly associated with a fetal sleep cycle but may result from any cause of central nervous system (CNS) depression, including fetal acidosis. It is an indirect measurement of uteroplacental function.

The patient is usually seated slightly tilted to the left to avoid supine hypotension. A Doppler ultrasound transducer and a tocodynamometer are used to monitor the fetal heart rate (FHR) and uterine activity simultaneously. Fetal movements should also be recorded during the test. (~65% of healthy fetuses will have a reactive NST at 28 weeks of gestation, 85% at 32 weeks and 95% at 34 weeks of gestation).

Results of NSTs are classified as *reactive* or *nonreactive*. NST is reactive or normal, if there are ≥2 FHR accelerations (each for 15 seconds and 15 beats above baseline) within a 20-minute period, associated with fetal movement.

Nonreactive NST may be present in fetal sleep, CNS depressants, anomalies of cardiovascular disease (CVS) and CNS, β-blockers, and chronic smoking.

- Advantage—easy to use and interpret
- Disadvantage—high false positive and negative rate

Cardiotocography

The CTG is a technique of recording the fetal heartbeat (cardio-) and the uterine contractions (-toco-) during pregnancy, typically in third trimester. The machine used to perform the monitoring is called a cardiotocograph, also known as an electronic fetal monitor (EFM). **Figure 1** shows a reactive CTG.

- Characteristics of CTG—baseline rate, baseline variability, accelerations, decelerations, and uterine activity (contractions)
- Baseline rate—normal 110–160 bpm, bradycardia <110 bpm, and tachycardia >160 bpm

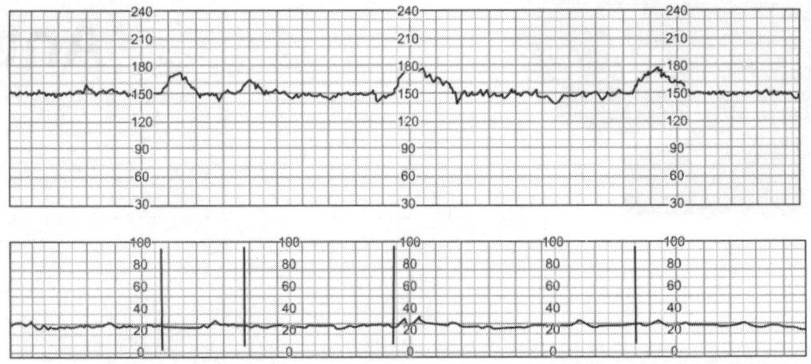

Fig. 1: Reactive cardiotocography (CTG).

- Baseline variability—maximum to minimum variation/ min, normal 5–25 bpm, increased >25 bpm, reduced <5 bpm, absent—straight line/sinusoidal
- Acceleration—transient increases in FHR of ≥15 bpm above the baseline, lasting ≥15 seconds. Two accelerations in 20 minutes are considered a reactive trace.
- Deceleration (periodic/episodic)—periodic refers to decelerations that are associated with contractions; episodic refers to those not associated with contraction. Four types of decelerations includes: (1) Early decelerations, (2) late deceleration, (3) variable deceleration, (4) prolonged deceleration. **Figures 2A to C** show different types of decelerations.
    1. Early deceleration begins at onset of the contraction and ends with the end of the contraction <30 seconds, caused by vagal stimulation due to head compression.
    2. Late decelerations are transitory decreases in FHR caused by utero placental insufficiency. It begins after onset of the peak/middle of contraction and ends after contraction is over.
    3. Variable decelerations are transitory decreases in FHR caused by umbilical cord compression (>30 seconds and <2 minutes), unrelated to uterine contractions (V- or U-shaped).
    4. Prolonged decelerations is decrease of FHR below the baseline of >15 bpm for longer ≥3 minutes.

Vibroacoustic or Fetal Acoustic Stimulation Test

The principle is to startle the fetus with a loud sound. Vibroacoustic stimulators are artificial larynxes, or an electric toothbrush held briefly to the maternal abdomen near the fetal head and generates sound pressure levels of approximately 80–100 decibels applied in 2–3 one-second bursts.

This essentially wakes a sleeping fetus, thereby changing its behavioral state.

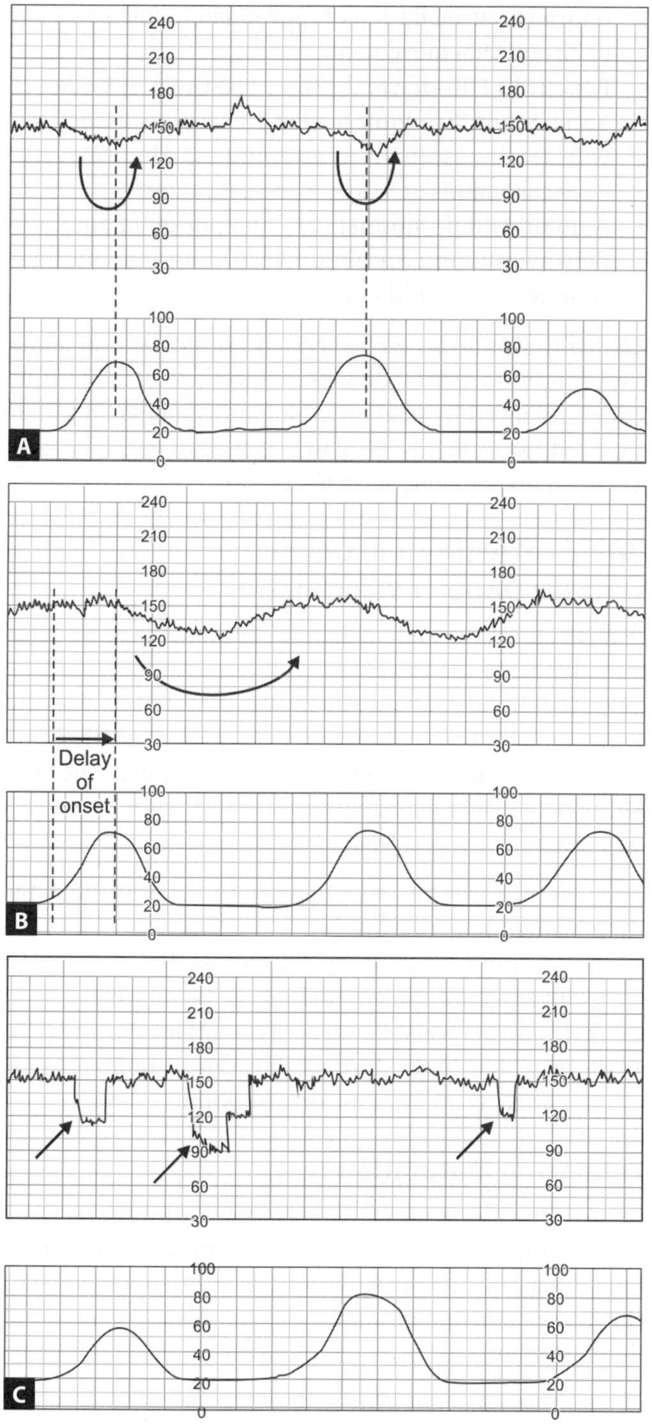

Figs. 2A to C: (A) Early deceleration; (B) Late deceleration; (C) Variable deceleration.

Fetuses that respond to vibroacoustic or fetal acoustic stimulation (VAS) with an acceleration on an NST or a startle response on a BPP have very low rates of death within one week of the test. The fetuses who are nonreactive even after VAS may be at increased risk and need immediate intervention.

Contraction Stress Test

The contraction stress test (CST), also referred to as the Oxytocin challenge test, more cumbersome to perform, more costly than the NST and also presents more risks. However, this may identify fetuses that are only marginally compromised by assessing their reserve when subjected to the stress of uterine contractions. Fetal oxygenation is worsened transiently by uterine contractions, if suboptimal oxygenation it will lead to the FHR pattern of late decelerations.

Contraction Stress Test Procedure

The patient is placed in semi fowler position at a 30–40-degree angle, with a slight tilt to the left to avoid supine hypotension. Baseline FHR and uterine tone are recorded on a cardiotocograph for 10–20 minutes. The test requires uterine contractions of 40–60 seconds with a frequency of 3 in 10 minutes for which Oxytocin is administered by an infusion pump at 0.5 mU/min, i.e., at least 3 contractions in 10 minutes and doubled every 20 minutes till required contractions occur (max 10 mU/min).

Interpretation of CST by the presence/absence of late FHR decelerations as follows:

- *Negative:* No late or significant variable decelerations
- *Positive:* Late decelerations following $\geq$50% of contractions.
- *Equivocal-suspicious:* Intermittent late decelerations or significant variable decelerations
- *Equivocal-hyperstimulatory:* FHR decelerations that occur in presence of contractions that are more frequent than every 2 minutes or last longer than 90 seconds.
- *Unsatisfactory:* $<$3 contractions in 10 minutes or a tracing that is not interpretable.

Contraindications due to risk of uterine hyperstimulation, it is contraindicated in patients who are at a high risk for preterm/premature labor, uterine rupture, or uterine bleeding.

Nipple Stimulation Test

Patient is advised to apply a warm moist towel to each breast for 5 minutes. If no uterine contractions occur then massage one nipple with palmar surface of fingers through her clothes for 2 minutes, stop for 5 minutes, and repeat if required. The cycle is repeated till adequate contractions are observed.

The test time is approximately 45 minutes. Hyperstimulation is avoided by intermittent stimulation.

Contraindications and interpretations are the same as for contraction stress test.

Biophysical Profile

Being an ultrasonographic assessment of fetal behavior, it requires more expensive equipment and more highly trained personnel than the other testing modalities. It is based on the concept that hypoxic fetuses lose certain behavioral parameters in the reverse order in which they were acquired in the course of fetal development. It evaluates indicators of chronic fetal hypoxia and placental function, such as amniotic fluid volume, in addition to more acute indicators, such as fetal breathing movements, and tone.

Five variables are assessed, two points are awarded for each, normal test has a maximum of 10 points.

Sequence of Fetal Deterioration

- Cardiac reactivity in nonstress test
- Fetal breathing
- Fetal movement
- Fetal tone
- Amniotic fluid decreases (chronic hypoxia)

Modified biophysical profile (MBP)—an alternative to the BPP is a combination of the NST and an assessment of amniotic fluid index (AFI). AFI <5 is considered abnormal.

TECHNIQUE OF MANNING'S BIOPHYSICAL PROFILE SCORING

- Fetal breathing—normal (score 2), at least one episode of >30 seconds in 30 minutes; and abnormal (score 0) if absent or no episode of >30 seconds in 30 minutes.
- Gross body—normal (2), at least three discrete body/limb movements in 30 minutes; and abnormal (0), up to two movements in 30 minutes.
- Fetal tone—normal (2), at least one episode of active extension to flexion of fetal limb/trunk, opening, and closing of hand; and abnormal (0), slow extension with return to partial flexion or movement in full extension or absent fetal movement.
- Reactive FHR—normal (2), at least two episodes of acceleration ≥15 bpm lasting 15 seconds associated with fetal movement in 30 minutes. Abnormal (0), <2 accelerations or <15 bpm in 30 minutes.
- Amniotic fluid—normal (2)—one pocket of amniotic fluid measuring 2 cm; abnormal (0)—no amniotic fluid volume or pocket <2 cm.

Clinically significant points: NST is an indicator of acute fetal condition and is the first one to be affected in BPP. This is followed by fetal breathing movements and then gross fetal movements. Fetal tone is the last to be affected. AFI is a marker of long-term fetal status.

Umbilical Artery and Ductus Venosus Doppler Velocimetry

Used to assess the hemodynamic components of vascular impedance, in umbilical artery in high-risk pregnancies only. The umbilical flow velocity waveform of a normally growing fetus has high-velocity forward diastolic flow, while in cases of IUGR, the umbilical artery diastolic flow is diminished and in extreme growth restriction, flow may be absent or even reversed.

Doppler ultrasound—not beneficial for routine fetal surveillance, main role in FGR.

- The umbilical artery systolic/diastolic (S/D) ratio >95th percentile for gestational age is abnormal.
- An absent or reverse flow is of value only in cases of IUGR.
- Reverse flow in the ductus venosus is an ominous sign and predicts intrauterine demise within 7 days.

Fetal Lung Maturation Tests

Fetal lung maturation tests predict the chances of developing respiratory distress syndrome (RDS). It includes assessment of surfactant lecithin/sphingomyelin (L/S) ratio, function of surfactant (shake test), or amniotic fluid turbidity.

Test for fetal lung maturity:

- Lecithin/sphingomyelin ratio
- Phosphatidylglycerol level
- Shake test ("bubble"/"foam" test)—formation of a stable ring of foam by shaking amniotic fluid mixed with ethanol.

RECOMMENDATIONS

- Women at high risk for stillbirth should undergo antepartum fetal surveillance.
- Initiation at 32–34 weeks of gestation is appropriate for most pregnancies that are at increased risk.
- When the clinical condition persists, a reassuring test should be repeated weekly or twice weekly until delivery.
- An abnormal NST or MBP usually should be further evaluated by a contraction stress test or a full BPP.
- Oligohydramnios requires close maternal or fetal surveillance.
- In absence of obstetric contraindications, delivery of the fetus with an abnormal test result may be attempted by induction of labor with continuous monitoring of the FHR and contractions.

  If repetitive late decelerations are observed, cesarean delivery generally is indicated.
- Umbilical artery Doppler velocimetry benefits pregnancies complicated by IUGR (FGR).
- Middle cerebral artery Doppler velocimetry should be considered an investigational approach to antepartum fetal surveillance.

SUGGESTED READING

1. Huddleston JF, Sutlift G, Robinson D. Contraction stress test by intermittent nipple stimulation. Obstet Gynecol. 1984; 63:669.
2. Manning FA. Biophysial profile screening in Nyhuis. In: Nijhuis J (Ed). Fetal Behaviour. New York: Oxford University Press; 1992. p. 241.
3. Spong CY. Danforth's Obstetrics and Gynecology, 9th edition. Philadelphia: Lippincott Williams and Wilkins. 2003. p. 159.

CHAPTER 8

Multiple Pregnancy

INTRODUCTION

Multiple pregnancy is a pregnancy with development of more than one fetus in utero at the same time. Simultaneous development of:

- Two fetuses—twins (most common)
- Three fetuses—triplets
- Four fetuses—quadruplets
- Five fetuses—quintuplets
- Six fetuses—sextuplets, etc.

Incidence of twin pregnancy: One in 60 pregnancies, highest in West Africa and lowest is in Asia. ↑Incidence due to two main factors:

1. Rise of infertility treatments (assisted reproductive technology) and ovulation-stimulating drugs
2. Shift toward an older maternal age at conception, naturally (∵↑Gonadotropins).

TYPES OF TWIN PREGNANCY

Twins will either be monozygotic or dizygotic.

- *Monozygotic/uniovular/identical twins:* Develop from fusion of one ovum and one spermatozoon, which after fertilization splits into two, of same sex, same genes, same blood group, and same physical features, e.g., eye and hair-color, ear shapes, and palm creases.
- *Dizygotic/binovular/fraternal/nonidentical twins:* Develop from two ova that are fertilized by two different spermatozoa during a single ovarian cycle, no more alike than any other brother or sister and of same or different sex.

ETIOLOGY

Exact cause is unknown.

- Race—frequency is highest among black race and lowest in Mongols.
- Heredity—more transmitted through the female (maternal side)
- Maternal age—↑ with advancing age, maximum between 30 and 35 years.
- Parity—increased especially from 5th pregnancy onward
- Iatrogenic—drugs for induction of ovulation.

Determination of Zygosity and Chorionicity

- *Zygosity* refers to degree of genetic similarity within each pair, monozygotic (identical)/dizygotic (nonidentical).
- *Chorionicity* refers to placenta, diagnosed by ultrasound preferably during first trimester.
- In monozygotic twins, twinning at different periods of division of embryonic plate:
    - If division within <72 hours, resulting embryos will have two separate placentae, chorions and amnions, i.e., dichorionic-diamniotic (DCDA).
    - If the division takes place between the 4th and 8th day, when chorion has already developed, i.e., monochorionic-diamniotic.
    - If the division takes place after >8th day of fertilization (when the amniotic cavity has already formed), i.e., monochorionic-monoamniotic (MCMA).
    - Rarely, division occurs after 2 weeks (development of embryonic disk) resulting in the formation of conjoined twins.
        - Thoracopagus (most common)
        - Pyopagus (posterior fusion)
        - Craniopagus (cephalic)
        - Ischiopagus (caudal)

DIAGNOSIS

- *History:*
    - Increased nausea and vomiting in early pregnancy
    - Cardiorespiratory embarrassment in later months (palpitations, shortness of breath)
    - Tendency of swelling of legs, varicose veins, and hemorrhoids is greater
    - Excessive fetal movements
    - Unusual rate of abdominal enlargement

- History of multiple pregnancy in the family (more on the maternal side)
- History of infertility treatment/ovulation inducing drugs

- *General examination:*
  - Signs of anemia
  - Unusual weight gain
  - Evidence of preeclampsia
- *Abdominal examination:*
  - *Inspection:*
    - Uterus barrel shaped
    - Abdomen unduly enlarged
  - *Palpation:*
    - Fundal height is > gestational age (GA)
    - Abdominal girth at level of umbilicus >100 cm at term
    - Palpation of multiple fetal parts and >3 fetal poles (cephalic/podalic)
  - *Auscultation:* Presence of two distinct fetal heart sounds located at separate spots (~10 cm) with a difference of at least 10 beats/min.

Diagnosis confirmed by ultrasound.

DIFFERENTIAL DIAGNOSIS OF ABDOMINAL FINDINGS OF UTERUS > GESTATIONAL AGE

- Multiple pregnancy
- Wrong dates
- Wrong examination
- Big fetus
- Polyhydramnios
- Pregnancy with uterine fibroids
- Pregnancy with an ovarian cyst
- Ascites with pregnancy
- Molar pregnancy
- Retention of urine (full bladder)

COMPLICATIONS

Maternal Complications

- *Antepartum complications of multiple pregnancy:* ↑Nausea and vomiting, anemia, preeclampsia, polyhydramnios, antepartum hemorrhage (APH), malpresentation, placenta previa, preterm labor, and mechanical distress
- *Intrapartum complications of multiple pregnancy:* Cord prolapse, premature rupture of membranes, prolonged labor, intrapartum bleeding, increased operative interference, and postpartum hemorrhage (PPH)
- *Postpartum complications of multiple pregnancy:* Subinvolution of the uterus, infection, and lactation failure.

Fetal Complications

Abortion, fetal growth restriction, preterm birth, cord prolapse, fetal abnormalities, discordant growth, vanishing twin, intrauterine death (IUD) of one fetus, twin-twin transfusion syndrome, locked twins, ↑perinatal mortality, and delayed second twin delivery (>60 minutes).

Other Complications

- Fetus papyraceous (compressus)—when one of the fetus dies early → dead fetus is flattened and compressed between membranes of the living fetus and the uterine wall, more common in monozygotic twins, usually discovered at delivery or earlier by ultrasonography (USG).
- Fetus acardius—one fetus without heart
- *Twin reversed arterial perfusion (TRAP):*
  - One twin presents without a well-defined cardiac structure and is kept alive through placental anastomoses to the circulatory system of the viable fetus.
  - It occurs only in twins or triplets.
- *Fetus-in-fetu (endoparasite):* A fetus may be lodged within another fetus (only in monozygotic twins).

MANAGEMENT

- First-trimester USG for GA determines chorionicity and amnionicity by number of placental masses, presence of amniotic membrane and membrane thickness, lambda [dichorionic twin (DCT)], or T-sign [monochorionic twin (MCT)].
- Estimate GA from the **largest baby** in a twin or triplet pregnancy to avoid the risk of estimating it from a baby with early growth pathology.
- If difficult to determine chorionicity, e.g., late booking, manage the pregnancy as a monochorionic pregnancy until proven otherwise.
- Apart from routine antenatal investigations, full blood count at 20–24 weeks to identify anemia, and repeat at 28 weeks as in routine antenatal care.
- Level-I and level-II scan, growth (discordant—difference of >20% in weight, >5% in head circumference,

>20 mm in abdominal circumference) scan, in MCT for twin-to-twin transfusion syndrome (TTTS) [oligohydramnios deepest vertical pocket (DVP) <2 cm and polyhydramnios DVP >10 cm]—from 16 weeks every fortnightly.

- Iron and Folic acid, Aspirin [low-dose Aspirin (LDA) if ≥2 risk factors for pregnancy-induced hypertension (PIH)], corticosteroids for fetal lung maturity (24–34 weeks) and $MgSO_4$ (<32 weeks) if likely to deliver in a week.
- Progesterone 200 mg vaginal pessary once a day at bedtime in twin/triplet pregnancy and cervical length of ≤25 mm till 34 weeks (or birth if sooner) [no intramuscular (IM) progesterone, arabin pessary, bed rest, cervical cerclage, and oral tocolytics to prevent preterm labor].
- Plan delivery for uncomplicated DCDA at 37 weeks, MCT at 36 weeks, triplets at 35 weeks and MCMA between 32 and 34 weeks, after steroid coverage. But if complicated then earlier delivery plan should be individualized.
- *Mode of delivery:* Uncomplicated twins (DCT/MCT) with first fetus in vertex → vaginal delivery with continuous electronic fetal monitoring (CEFM). Lower segment cesarean section (LSCS) → if any complications [discordant growth, TTTS, TRAP, twin anemia-polycythemia sequence (TAPS), and single fetal demise], triplets, and MCMA twins
- Vaginal delivery—first stage—bed rest, analgesics, and electronic fetal monitoring
- Per vaginal examination rule out cord prolapse soon after rupture of membrane, intravenous (IV) line, cross-matched blood
- Delivery of first baby—liberal episiotomy, forceps delivery if needed, no Ergometrine, clamp cord at two places and cut between, leave at least 8–10 cm of cord, and hand over the baby
- After delivery of first baby check lie/presentation/size/FHS of 2nd baby by clinically/USG, per vaginal examination to confirm abdominal findings, and rule out cord prolapse
- Second baby longitudinal—Syntocinon drip → fix presenting part → artificial rupture of membrane, exclude cord prolapse, fetal monitoring, vertex—low down → forceps, high up → rule out cephalopelvic disproportion (CPD)/hydrocephalous → internal podalic version (IPV) followed by breech extraction/ventouse; breech → breech extraction
- Second baby transverse—external cephalic version (ECV) → longitudinal → cephalic/podalic; if fails → IPV followed by breech extraction
- Urgent delivery of second twin—severe intrapartum bleeding, Ergometrine given with delivery of first baby, cord prolapse, fetal distress, first baby delivered under GA
- *Active management of the third stage of labor (AMTSL):* In a vaginal birth, active management—10 IU of Oxytocin by IM injection immediately after the birth of the last baby and before the cord is clamped and cut. In a cesarean section—5 IU of Oxytocin by slow IV injection immediately after the birth of the last baby and before the cord is clamped and cut.

SUGGESTED READING

1. ACOG. (2021). Multifetal gestations twin triplet and higher-order multifetal pregnancies. [online] Available from https://www.acog.org/clinical/clinical-guidance/practice-bulletin/articles/2021/06/multifetal-gestations-twin-triplet-and-higher-order-multifetal-pregnancies [Last accessed September, 2024].
2. NICE. (2019). Twin and triplet pregnancy—NICE guideline [NG137]. [online] Available from https://www.nice.org.uk/guidance/ng137 [Last accessed September, 2024].

CHAPTER 9

Hypertensive Disorders of Pregnancy

Table 1 shows the classification of hypertensive disorders in pregnancy.

PREECLAMPSIA: RISK FACTORS (NICE)

- High risk if **any one** of the following—Obstetric history of pregnancy-induced hypertension/preeclampsia (PIH/PE), chronic kidney disease (CKD), autoimmune disease systemic lupus erythematosus/antiphospholipid antibody (SLE/APLA), type 1 or type 2 diabetes mellitus (DM), chronic hypertension (HTN)
- Moderate risk if **two or more**—nulliparity, age ≥40 years, pregnancy interval >10 years, ≥body mass index (BMI) 35 kg/m^2 at first visit, F/H of PE, and multiple pregnancy.

Advise Aspirin 75–150 mg daily from 12 weeks until delivery, if above risks are present.

Box 1 shows gestosis score ≥3 - high risk for hypertensive disorders of pregnancy.

TABLE 1: Classification of hypertensive disorders in pregnancy.

Gestational hypertension	• Hypertension for first time during pregnancy • No proteinuria • Blood pressure returns to normal before 12 weeks postpartum
Preeclampsia and eclampsia	• Hypertension diagnosed after 20 weeks' gestation • Proteinuria • May have other signs or symptoms of preeclampsia • Presence of features of severity in the absence of proteinuria • Eclampsia when accompanied by seizures that cannot be attributed to other causes
Preeclampsia superimposed on chronic hypertension	• New-onset proteinuria in hypertensive women after 20 weeks' gestation • Worsening or resistant hypertension (especially acutely or development of signs/symptoms of the severe end-of-the-disease spectrum in women with hypertension and proteinuria before 20 weeks' gestation
Chronic hypertension	• Hypertension before pregnancy • Hypertension diagnosed before 20 weeks' gestation, not attributable to gestational trophoblastic disease or multiple pregnancy • Hypertension first diagnosed after 20 weeks' gestation and persistent beyond 12 weeks postpartum

BOX 1: Gestosis score risk calculation.

Mild-risk factors (score 1):
- Age older than 35 years
- Age younger than 19 years
- Maternal anemia
- Obesity (BMI >30)
- Primigravida
- Short duration of paternity (cohabitation)
- Woman born as small for GA
- PCOS
- Interpregnancy interval >5 years
- Conceived with ART (IVF/ICSI)
- MAP >85
- Chronic vascular disease (dyslipidemia)
- Excessive weight gain during pregnancy

Moderate-risk factors (score 2):
- Maternal hypothyroidism
- Family history of preeclampsia
- GDM
- Multiple pregnancy
- Obesity (BMI >35)
- Hypertensive disease during previous pregnancy

Severe-risk factors (score 3):
- Pregestational DM
- Chronic hypertension
- Mental disorder
- Inherited/acquired thrombophilia
- Maternal chronic kidney disease
- Autoimmune disease (SLE/APLAS/RA)
- Pregnancy with ART (**OD** or surrogacy)

(APLAS: antiphospholipid **antibody**; ART: assisted reproductive technology; BMI: body mass index; DM: diabetes mellitus; GA: gestational age; ICSI: intracytoplasmic sperm injection; IVF: in vitro fertilization; MAP: mean arterial pressure; OD: oocyte donation; PCOS: polycystic ovary syndrome; RA: rheumatoid arthritis; SLE: systemic lupus erythematosus)

DIAGNOSTIC CRITERIA FOR PREECLAMPSIA

- *Blood pressure (BP):*
  - Systolic BP (SBP) ≥140 mm Hg and or diastolic BP (DBP) ≥90 mm Hg on two occasions 4 hours apart after 20 weeks of gestation with previous normal BP
  - SBP ≥160 mm Hg and or DBP ≥110 mm Hg (severe HTN) can be confirmed within a short interval (10–15 minutes) to facilitate timely antihypertensive therapy
- *Proteinuria:*
  - ≥ 300 mg/24-hour urine collection or
  - Spot urine protein/creatinine ratio (UPCR) ≥30 mg/mmol, albumin:creatinine ≥8 mg/mmol
  - Dipstick of more than or equal to 2+ (if quantitative methods unavailable)
- Or in the absence of proteinuria, new-onset HTN with any of the following:
  - Thrombocytopenia
  - *Impaired liver function:* Elevated liver enzymes (twice normal), severe persistent right upper quadrant pain unresponsive to medication and no alternative diagnosis
  - Renal insufficiency (serum creatinine ≥1.1 mg/dL or doubling in absence of renal disease)
  - Pulmonary edema
  - New-onset headache unresponsive to medication and no alternative diagnosis
  - Visual disturbances

PATHOGENESIS

In early pregnancy, cytotrophoblast infiltrates decidual portion of spiral arteries but fails to invade myometrial portion thus vessels remain narrow, resulting in placental underperfusion/hypoxia/ischemia which releases antiangiogenic factors in maternal circulation that alter systemic endothelial function and causes HTN and other organ dysfunction.

Predictors of Preeclampsia

First trimester ↑ soluble Flt-1 (sFlt-1): Vascular endothelial growth factor (VEGF) or increases Flt-1: Placental growth factor (PlGF), positive roll-over test, low mid-trimester mean arterial pressure (MAP), persistence of diastolic notch in uterine artery Doppler >24 weeks, PlGF between 20 weeks and 36^{+6} weeks in PIH/chronic HTN or suspicion of PE.

Management of Preeclampsia

Labetalol/Nifedipine/Methyldopa, aim for BP ≤135/85 mm Hg, full blood count, liver function tests (LFTs), renal function test (RFT) at presentation and then twice weekly, ultrasonography (USG) Obs and nonstress test (NST), if controlled then plan delivery >37 completed weeks (either full Pre-eclampsia Integrated Estimate of RiSk for mothers (PIERS) (anytime) or Prediction models for Risks of complications in Early-onset Pre-eclampsia (PREP)-S (<34 weeks) validated risk prediction models to guide decisions about the most appropriate place of care (such as the need for in utero transfer) and thresholds for intervention.

Timing of birth in women with preeclampsia <34 weeks intravenous (IV) Magnesium sulfate and antenatal corticosteroids, if inability to control maternal BP despite using ≥3 classes of antihypertensives in appropriate doses, maternal pulse oximetry <90%, progressive deterioration in liver function, renal function, hemolysis, or platelet count; ongoing neurological features, such as severe intractable headache, repeated visual scotomata, or eclampsia, placental abruption, reversed end-diastolic flow in the umbilical artery Doppler velocimetry, a nonreassuring cardiotocograph, or stillbirth.

From 34 to 36 weeks plus 6 days: Consider a course of antenatal corticosteroids.

37 weeks onwards: Initiate birth within 24–48 hours.

PREECLAMPSIA WITH SEVERE FEATURES (ANY OF THESE FINDINGS)

- SBP ≥160 mm Hg and/or DBP ≥110 mm Hg on two occasion 15 minutes apart while patient is resting.
- Thrombocytopenia
- Impaired liver functions
- Renal insufficiency (serum creatinine ≥1.1 mg/dL or doubling in absence of renal disease)
- Pulmonary edema
- New-onset headache unresponsive to medication and not accounted for by any alternative diagnosis
- Visual disturbances

Management of Severe Preeclampsia

Investigations:

- Complete blood count (CBC) with platelet count
- RFT: Urea and creatinine
- *LFT*: Bilirubin, liver enzymes, and serum protein

- Coagulation profile
- Lactate dehydrogenase (LDH) (optional), urine dipstick/boiling after acetic acid/urinary protein to creatinine ratio (UPCR)
- Fundus examination
- Electrocardiography (ECG)
- NST, USG obs

Management:

- Start an IV line in casualty, IV fluids—80 mL/h unless there are other ongoing losses.
- Monitor BP, respiratory rate SpO_2, deep tendon reflexes, fetal heart rate, and auscultate lung bases—hourly
- Injection Dexamethasone 6 mg intramuscular (IM) 12 hourly for four doses if gestation <34 weeks
- If SBP remains ≥160 mm Hg or if DBP remains ≥110 mm Hg administer antihypertensives as per emergent management protocol.
- Give injection Magnesium sulfate, if BP is persistently high or in women with signs symptoms of impending eclampsia.
- Catheterize the bladder.
- Maintain strict input output chart.

Severe Hypertension

Systolic BP ≥160 mm Hg or DBP ≥110 mm Hg.

Hypertensive emergency:

- Persistent, severe HTN that can occur antepartum, intrapartum, or postpartum
- Two severe BP values (≥160/110 mm Hg) taken 15–60 minutes apart

First-line therapies:

- IV Labetalol
- IV Hydralazine
- Oral Nifedipine

Flowchart 1 shows the algorithm of Labetalol.

Antihypertensive should be initiated as early as possible in PE with severe features, and within 30-60 minutes. Continue BP monitoring every 15 minutes for 2 hours after stabilization then every 30 minutes for 1 hour. Then every hour if in labor or 4 hours if not in labor. Maintain BP ≤130/85 mm Hg. Once BP is controlled switch to oral drugs. Tablet Labetalol 200 mg TDS or capsule Nifedipine 10–20 mg BD or TDS.

- *Eclampsia:* Eclampsia is defined as the development of seizures that cannot be attributed to other causes and/or unexplained coma during pregnancy or puerperium in a woman with preeclampsia.
- *Impending eclampsia:* Persistent headache—occipital or frontal, visual disturbances—blurred vision or photophobia, restlessness and agitation, epigastric and/or right upper quadrant pain, nausea/vomiting, oliguria, laboratory evidence of disseminated intravascular coagulation (DIC).

Management

The management of eclampsia involves six stages:

Flowchart 1: Labetalol algorithm.

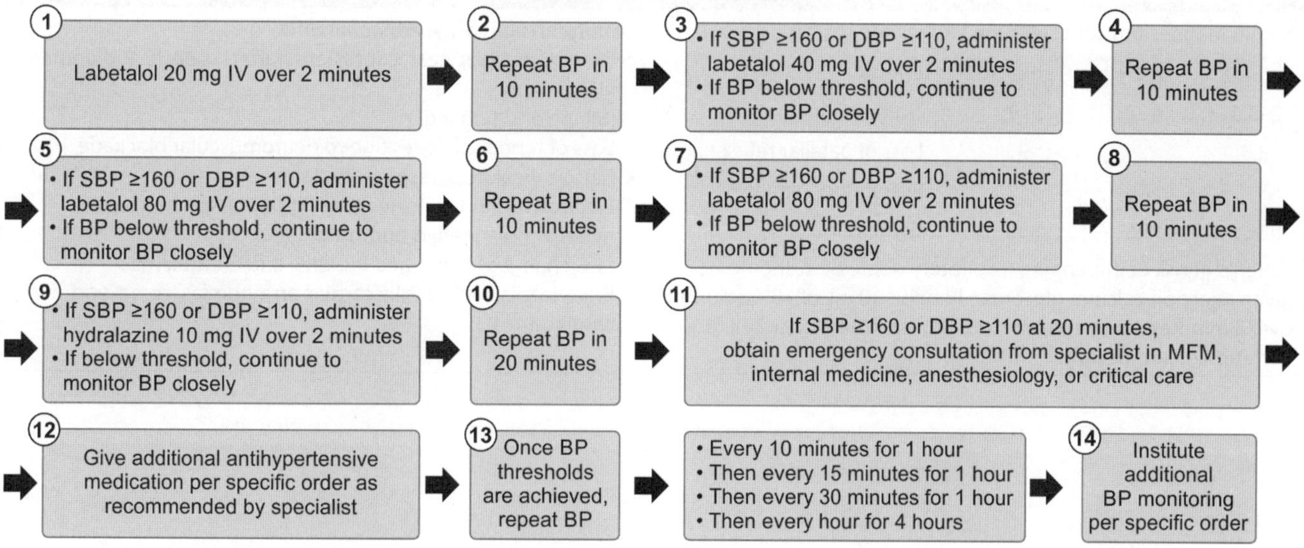

(BP: blood pressure; DBP: diastolic BP; IV: intravenous; MFM: maternal–fetal medicine; SBP: systolic BP)

1. Clearing the airway
2. Controlling seizures
3. Controlling the BP
4. General care and monitoring
5. Delivering the baby
6. Postpartum monitoring to prevent further convulsions and other complications.

Take a quick history and perform rapid evaluation of general condition:
- Call for help
- Check airway, if she is breathing, give oxygen at 4–6 L per minute by mask or nasal cannula. If not breathing, call anesthetist, assist ventilation using an Ambu bag and mask or intubate
- Secure IV line, send investigations and blood for cross matching
- Catheterize once patient is stable
- Check BP, pulse rate (PR), RR, temperature, pallor, icterus, cyanosis, pedal edema, and SpO_2
- Perform a cardiovascular system (CVS), respiratory, central nervous system (CNS) and obstetric examination as detailed below
- Give loading dose of Magnesium sulfate
- Antihypertensives as per emergent therapy
- Shift to high-dependency unit (HDU) once stable and start induction of labor
- *Mode of delivery:* Induction of labor is reasonable, do early ARM
- Cesarean delivery should be individualized based on obstetric indication.
- Aim to deliver within 6 to 12 hours for eclampsia

WHO recommends the *Pritchard regimen* for Magnesium sulfate, which is as follows:
- *Loading dose:* Magnesium sulfate 4 g (20 mL of 20% solution) IV slowly over 20 minutes PLUS 10 g IM-5 g (10 mL of 50% solution) with 1 mL of 2% Lignocaine in the same syringe deep in upper outer quadrant of each buttock.
- *Maintenance dose:* 5 g Magnesium sulfate (50% solution) together with 1 mL Lignocaine 2% in the same syringe every 4 hours into alternate buttock.
    - Continue the treatment with Magnesium sulfate for 24 hours after delivery or last convulsion, which ever is later.
    - Observations which must be recorded before giving repeat doses of $MgSO_4$. RR, patellar reflexes, and urinary output

Repeat doses of $MgSO_4$ must be withheld or delayed, if:
- RR is <14 breaths/min.
- Patellar reflexes are absent.
- Urinary output is <30 mL/h over preceding 4 hours.

In cases of respiratory arrest: Give Calcium gluconate 1 g (10 mL of 10% solution) IV slowly until respiration is satisfactory, assist ventilation using mask and bag, anesthetic apparatus, or intubation.

TABLE 2: Magnesium toxicity.

Serum Magnesium concentration and related toxicity

mmol/L	*mEq/L*	*mg/dL*	*Effects*
2–3.5	4–7	5–9	Therapeutic
>3.5	>7	>9	Loss of patellar reflex
>5	>10	>12	Respiratory paralysis
>12	>25	>30	Cardiac arrest

Patients at risk of impending respiratory depression should be given injection calcium gluconate IV bolus 10 mL of 10% solution over 3 minutes along with injection furosemide IV to accelerate excretion of Magnesium

Symptoms/signs of hypermagnesemia:
- Drowsiness, dizziness, confusion, slurred speech, and double vision
- Itching and tingling
- Loss of tendon reflexes due to neuromuscular blockade
- Muscle weakness, respiratory depression
- Electrolyte/fluid abnormalities (hypophosphatemia), hyperosmolar dehydration)
- ECG changes (prolonged PR, QRS, and QT intervals)
- Bradycardia, tachycardia cardiac arrhythmias, coma, and cardiac arrest

TABLE 3: Drugs and doses for severe hypertension in pregnancy.

Injection Labetalol	• 10–20 mg slow IV bolus over 2 minutes → 40 mg • 80 mg → 80 mg → (BP every 20–30 minutes) • Maximum of 220 mg can be given or if target BP <160/100 mm Hg is achieved • *For infusion*: 1–2 mg/min	• Avoid in asthma, congestive heart failure, heart block, and bradycardia • *Adverse effects:* Bradycardia • Hypotension • Fetal bradycardia
Injection Hydralazine	• 5 mg IV or IM, then 5–10 mg every 20–30 minutes (max dose 20 mg) • *For infusion:* 0.5–10.0 mg/h	*Adverse effects:* Hypotension, headache, flushing, tachycardia, dizziness, and abnormal fetal heart rate tracing
Tablet Nifedipine	Only tablets recommended: 10 mg stat per oral, repeat every 20 minutes	*Adverse effects:* Flushing headache, dizziness, nausea hypotension, tachycardia, and myocardial infarction
Nitroglycerine drip	*Nitroglycerin (NTG) drip:* • Injection NTG 5 mL (25 mg) + 45 mL NS = 50 mL • Desired dose: 1 µg/min • (Available dose: 25 mg)	Hypotension, dizziness, flushing, and headache

Table 2 shows Magnesium toxicity levels and its signs and symptoms.

Table 3 shows antihypertensives in severe hypertension.

SUGGESTED READING

1. Gestational Hypertension and Preeclampsia: ACOG Practice Bulletin: 202. Obst Gynecol. 2019;133(1):e1-17.
2. Gestational Hypertension and Preeclampsia: ACOG Practice Bulletin Summary, Number 222. Obstet Gynecol. 2020;135(6):1492-5.
3. Misra R. Ian Donald Practical Obstetrics Problems, 9th edition. India: Wolters Kluwer India; 2020.
4. NICE. (2019). Hypertension in Pregnancy: Diagnosis and management. NICE Guideline N133; 2019. [online] Available from https://www.nice.org.uk/guidance/ng133 [Last accessed September, 2024].

CHAPTER 10

Antepartum Hemorrhage

DEFINITION

Bleeding from or into female genital tract after the period of viability (24^{+0} weeks in developed and 28^{+0} weeks in developing countries) but before the delivery of baby (includes first stage of labor also). Incidence—3–5%.

CLASSIFICATION

- *Placental bleeding:* Placenta previa and abruptio placenta
- *Extraplacental bleeding: Genital* infections (TV), *lacerations,* cervical lesions—erosion, polyp, growth, cancer, varicosities—vulval/vaginal, and vasa previa (rare).

Placenta Previa

When placenta implanted partially or totally on lower uterine segment (LUS). "Low lying" when placental edge <20 mm from internal os, term "placenta praevia" is used when placenta lies directly over internal os:

- *Incidence:* 1:200
- *Risk factors:* Previous placenta previa, previous lower segment cesarean section (LSCS), history of termination of pregnancy, multiparity, advanced maternal age (>40 years), multiple pregnancy, smoking; deficient endometrium due to presence or history of—uterine scar, endometritis, manual removal of placenta, curettage, submucous fibroid; assisted conception
- *Etiology:* Implantation of fertilized ovum in the isthmus—area between anatomical and histological internal os, decidua capsularis develops into chorion or large placenta (e.g., multiple pregnancy)
- *Mechanism of bleeding:* A shearing force develops between inelastic placenta and LUS, as the LUS grows, leading to placental separation (maternal blood)
- *Clinical picture:* Painless, causeless, and recurrent bleeding ± warning hemorrhages
- *Signs:* G/E—according to severity of bleeding ± anemia, tachycardia, and hypotension
- *P/A:* Uterus soft and nontender, associated with malpresentation or high floating head. If previous scan shows a low placenta, high presenting part on abdominal examination, or bleeding, i.e., painless. Digital vaginal examination should not be performed until an ultrasound has excluded placenta previa, except in theatre (double set up), but sterile speculum examination done to rule out local cause as well as cervical dilatation. Active treatment done during labor and in case of severe bleeding.
- *Investigation:*
  - Full blood count (FBC), ABO and Rh (crossmatch blood), coagulation profile, liver function test (LFT), renal function test (RFT), ultrasound, and cardiotocogram (CTG), if RhD-negative Kleihauer test for fetomaternal hemorrhage (FMH) to calculate dose of anti-D immunoglobulin (Ig).
  - About 18–20 weeks anomaly/level-II scan can identify placenta previa or a low-lying placenta. Placenta previa—if placenta is directly over internal os, and low-lying placenta if placental edge <20 mm from the internal os on transabdominal sonography or transvaginal sonography (TAS or TVS).
  - If placenta low lying or previa on routine anomaly scan, a follow-up ultrasonography (USG) including TVS recommended at 32 weeks to diagnose persistent low-lying placenta and/or placenta previa (TVS > TAS). Also short cervical length on TVS < 34 weeks of gestation increases risk of preterm emergency delivery and massive hemorrhage at cesarean section (CS).
  - In asymptomatic persistent low-lying placenta or placenta previa at 32 weeks, TAS/TVS should be done at ~36 weeks of gestation to decide mode of delivery.
- *Complications:*
  - *Maternal:*
    - *During pregnancy:* Antepartum hemorrhage (APH), malpresentation/unstable lie/high-floating head, and preterm labor (PTL)

- During labor: Bleeding, uterine inertia, ↑chance of LSCS, and postpartum hemorrhage (PPH)
- During puerperium: Puerperal sepsis and subinvolution

- *Fetal:* Prematurity, fetal distress due to anemia and hypoxia, cord prolapse, and perinatal mortality 10–15%

- *Management:*
  - Hospitalization, multidisciplinary team (MDT)—obstetric unit, anesthetist, blood bank, intensive care unit (ICU), neonatal ICU (NICU), and pediatrician. A single course of antenatal corticosteroid should be given between 34^{+0} and 35^{+6} weeks as they are at higher risk of preterm birth. Tocolysis for women presenting with symptomatic placenta previa or a low-lying placenta may be considered for 48 hours to facilitate administration of antenatal corticosteroids. If delivery is indicated based on maternal or fetal concerns, tocolysis should **not** be used in an attempt to prolong gestation.
  - *Delivery:* Late preterm (34^{+0}–36^{+6} weeks) delivery for placenta previa/low-lying placenta with history of bleeding per **vaginum** or other risk factors for preterm delivery; and for uncomplicated placenta previa, delivery should be considered between 36^{+0} and 37^{+0} weeks of gestation.
  - *CS:* Vertical skin and/or uterine incisions if fetus is in transverse lie to avoid placenta, especially <28 weeks. If placenta transected during uterine incision, the umbilical cord should be clamped immediately after delivery of fetus to avoid fetal blood loss. If pharmacological measures fail to control hemorrhage, initiate intrauterine tamponade, and/or surgical hemostatic techniques sooner rather than later. Interventional radiological techniques should also be urgently employed where possible. If medical and surgical interventions are not effective in controlling hemorrhage, early recourse to hysterectomy is recommended.

Accidental Hemorrhage (Abruptio Placenta)

- *Definition:* Separation of normally situated placenta after period of viability (24^{+0} weeks developed and 28^{+0} weeks developing).
- *Risk factors:* Previous abruptio, ↑maternal age, multiparity, low-socioeconomic status, ↓body mass index (BMI), preeclampsia, fetal growth restriction, nonvertex presentations, polyhydramnios, multiple pregnancy, pregnancy after assisted reproductive technology (ART), intrauterine infection, preterm labor or preterm premature rupture of membrane (PTPROM), abdominal trauma (accidental and domestic violence), smoking, drug misuse (Cocaine and Amphetamines), and thrombophilia.
- *Incidence:* About 1%, recurrence: 10–15%
- *Etiology:*
  - *Toxemia:* Spasm of blood vessel leading to capillary anoxia and endothelial disruption, degeneration, rupture, or bleeding. Possible role of membrane protein RCAS1 (receptor-binding cancer antigen on Siso cells) that maintains immune tolerance in pregnancy.
  - *Nontoxemia: Placental* (*circumvallate* placenta)/cord abnormalities, blunt abdominal trauma, external cephalic version, traction on cord, increased intrauterine pressure as in case of polyhydramnios leading to sudden rupture of membranes, folate deficiency, and rapid decompression of uterus after delivery of first twin.
    - *Uteroplacenta apoplexy (Couvelaire's uterus) coagulation defect pathology:* Blood dissects into layers of myometrium due to degeneration and splitting of decidua basalis and hematoma formation. Besides thromboplastin enters directly into maternal circulation through lacerations in decidual layers resulting in coagulopathy.
- *Investigation:* ABO and Rh, FBC, LFT, RFT, coagulation profile, urine analysis, and USG (miss 50%)
- *Diagnosis:* Purely clinical:
  - *Symptoms:* Abdominal cramps, backache, may/may not associated with vaginal bleeding—dark red with/without clots.
  - *Sign:* G/E—hypertensive (or shock) unrelated to amount of blood loss. Pulse↑, blood pressure (BP) ↓, ± temperature subnormal, edema due to preeclampsia, ecchymosis, or petechiae if disseminated intravascular coagulation (DIC)
    - *P/A:* Large uterus tense, tender and rigid with/without tetanic contractions (severe cases) or may be irritable with/without contractions (nonsevere cases), fetal heart sound (FHS) not heard/signs of distress

- *P/V:* No/mild bleeding with or without dilated cervix
- *D/D:* Rupture uterus, retroperitoneal hematoma, rectus sheath hematoma, acute polyhydramnios, acute pyelonephritis, and nonobstetric causes of acute abdomen

- *Management of placenta abruption—MDT:* Principle of management:
  - Early delivery (50% of abruption present in labor)
  - Intravenous (IV) line and intake/output (I/O) charting
  - Adequate blood transfusion, fresh frozen plasma (FFP)/cryoprecipitate, and platelets
  - Detailed maternal and electronic fetal monitoring (EFM)
  - Coagulation profile (30% develop DIC)
  - CS—distressed baby, severe bleeding, and alive baby not in advanced labor. Perinatal mortality rate is 15–20%.
  - Vaginal delivery—low gestation and dead baby, cervix is fully dilated (ventouse delivery).
  - Expectant management—small abruption, well mother, and fetus, if the gestational age is <34 weeks, give steroids. No tocolysis

Time taken to achieve delivery depends on rate of the bleeding, rate of change in clotting studies, and clinical condition of the mother and fetus.

- CTG twice/day
- Serial U/S and umbilical artery Doppler waveform
- No conservative after 38 weeks of gestation
- Anti-D if the mother is Rhesus negative
- Anticipate PPH
- In cases of previous CS, discuss hysterectomy
- In massive blood loss or a major abruption, DIC should be ruled out by clotting studies and platelet count urgently, and advice from a hematologist. Up to 4 units FFP and 10 units of cryoprecipitate can be given whilst awaiting the results of the coagulation studies.

- *Prognosis:*
  - *Maternal mortality*—1%, due to DIC, PPH and shock, acute renal failure (ARF), sepsis; depends on extent of abruptio, coagulation defect, and degree of uteroplacental apoplexy along with time of presentation and rapidity of management
  - *Fetal mortality*—100% in severe, 30–50% in revealed type
- *Complications of antepartum hemorrhage:*
  - Premature delivery
  - Fetal distress and death
  - Hemorrhagic shock
  - ARF due to acute tubular or cortical necrosis
  - DIC (release of tissue thromboplastin)
  - Uterine atony (couvelaire uterus)
  - PPH

SUGGESTED READING

1. Cunningham F, Leveno KJ, Dashe JS, Hoffman BL, Spong CY, Casey BM. Williams Obstetrics, 26 edition. Philadelphia: McGraw Hill; 2022.
2. Dalal A. D C Dutta's Textbook of Gynaecology and Textbook of Obstetrics. J Obstet Gynaecol India. 2021;66(4):303-4.
3. Misra R. Ian Donald's Practical Obstetrical Problems, 9th edition. India: Wolters Kluwer; 2020.
4. RCOG. (2011). Antepartum Haemorrhage (Green-top Guideline No. 63). [online] Available from https://www.rcog.org.uk/guidance/browse-all-guidance/green-top-guidelines/antepartum-haemorrhage-green-top-guideline-no-63/#:~:text=Summary,are%20not%20the%20most%20common [Last accessed September, 2024].
5. RCOG. (2018). Placenta Praevia and Placenta Accreta: Diagnosis and Management (Green-top Guideline No. 27a). [online] Available from https://www.rcog.org.uk/guidance/browse-all-guidance/green-top-guidelines/placenta-praevia-and-placenta-accreta-diagnosis-and-management-green-top-guideline-no-27a/ [Last accessed September, 2024].

CHAPTER 11

Rh Negative Pregnancy

INTRODUCTION

Landsteiner and Wiener, 1940 discovered in human red blood cell (RBC). Incidence—1% in China (nil—Japan), 100% in Basques, 15–17% in American and European whites, and 5–10% in India.

Genotype—"D" most potent antigen; D+ve is Rh positive and D-ve is Rh negative. Individual having DD homozygous accounts for 65%, individual having Dd heterozygous for 35%. Genetic locus is on the short arm of chromosome 1.

RH ALLOIMMUNIZATION (ISOIMMUNIZATION)

Production of immune antibodies in an individual in response to foreign red cell antigen derived from another individual of same species, provided, the first one lacks the antigen.

- *Two stages:* (1) Sensitization and (2) immunization
- *Methods:* (1) Mismatched blood transfusion and (2) pregnancy—Rh-ve women carrying Rh+ve fetus
- *Types of antibodies:* Immunoglobulin M (IgM)—first to appear, complete antibody, larger molecule, unable to cross placental barrier, not harmful to fetus, and agglutinates RBC containing D when suspended in saline. IgG appears later, incomplete antibody, small molecule, it crosses the placental barrier and damages the fetus, and agglutinates RBC with D, only when suspended in 20% albumin.

Not all at risk Rh-ve gets isoimmunized due to ABO incompatibility, e.g., if mother—O, father—A/B/AB, inborn inability to respond to Rh antigen stimulus, immunological nonresponder, variable antigenic stimulus, insufficient placental transfer of fetal antigens/maternal Ab formation, and volume of fetal blood entering in maternal circulation.

DURING PREGNANCY

Fetomaternal bleed increases in frequency and size with advancing gestation, in first trimester→ (3%) 0.03 mL which increases in third trimester → (45%) 25 mL. In spontaneous abortion <1% (0.1 mL), ↑in induced abortion to 20–25%. ↑ Risk—MTP, chorionic villus sampling (CVS), amniocentesis, ectopic, molar pregnancy, cordocentesis, antepartum hemorrhage (APH), external cephalic version (ECV), trauma, delivery, manual removal of placenta, and cesarean section (CS).

Fetal Affection by Rh Antibody

If Rh-ve fetus no effect on it. If fetus is Rh+ve, depending on degree of agglutination and destruction of fetal RBC; three types of hemolytic diseases are:

1. *Hydrops fetalis*—most serious, excessive destruction of fetal RBC → severe anemia, tissue anoxia, metabolic acidosis → affects fetal heart, brain, and placenta → placental hyperplasia, hypoproteinemia leading to generalized edema, ascites, hydrothorax, cardiac failure and fetal death, and baby—stillborn/macerated/neonatal demise. Diagnosis—mother Rh-ve, Rh antibody present, polyhydramnios, history of affection of baby due to hemolytic disease. USG—edema in skin, scalp, pleural, pericardial effusion, and straight X-ray abdomen show "Buddha" position of fetus with halo around head (due to scalp edema), large placenta.
2. *Icterus gravis neonatorum*—lesser form of fetal hemolysis, baby born alive without features of jaundice, but develops within 24 hours of birth. During pregnancy, unconjugated bilirubin excreted by placenta, fetal lungs, and skin into amniotic fluid. As soon as the cord is clamped—with continuing hemolysis, bilirubin increases and as liver is premature, it fails to conjugate it. If bilirubin >20 mg/dL—kernicterus.
3. *Congenital anemia of newborn:* Mildest form of hemolysis, anemia develops slowly, within first few weeks of life but no jaundice develops, RBC destruction continues up to 6 weeks, after which no maternal antibody is available for hemolysis. Hepatosplenomegaly, due to extramedullary erythropoiesis.

CLINICAL FEATURES

Mother—preeclampsia, polyhydramnios, macrocosmic baby, hypofibrinogenemia, and PPH; "maternal mirror syndrome" or "Ballantyne syndrome"—triad of fetal hydrops, placental edema and maternal edema.

PREVENTION OF RH ISOIMMUNIZATION

Avoid mismatched blood transfusion, no Rh+ve blood to Rh-ve, prevent/minimize fetomaternal bleed, during lower segment CS (LSCS)—avoid blood spillage in peritoneal cavity, no routine MRP, prophylactic Ergometrine should be avoided, amniocentesis should be done after placental localization, avoid forcible attempt during ECV, refrain from abdominal palpation in abruption placenta, and gentle MRP.

Active immunization → Rh anti-D immunoglobulin IM to mother during pregnancy at 28 weeks and after childbirth, CVS or amniocentesis, during ECV, surgical termination of pregnancy or ectopic, APH, and intrauterine device (IUD).

According to NICE—do not offer anti-D immunoglobulin prophylaxis to women who receive solely medical management for an ectopic pregnancy or miscarriage or have a threatened miscarriage or have a complete miscarriage or have a pregnancy of unknown location (2012). Also do not use a Kleihauer test for quantifying fetomaternal hemorrhage (2012).

Rh Anti-D immunoglobulin—mode of action (antibody-mediated immune suppression): It blocks Rh antigen of fetal cells, Ab-coated fetal RBCs removed by RES-spleen, lymph nodes; central inhibition interferes with Ab production by B-cells, Timing should be administered within 72 hours of delivery, prophylactic one dose at 28 weeks (repeat + after delivery if baby blood group Rh+ve), and dose—300 μg (for 30 mL fetal blood/15 mL fetal RBC).

Antenatal Investigation

First antenatal visit—ABO and Rh of every pregnant women, if Rh-ve—husband's Rh typing, if husband is Rh +ve → husband's genotype—homozygous (100% affected)/heterozygous (50% affected). If fetal blood group by noninvasive prenatal testing test (NIPT) (-ve routine ANC), +ve antibody detection by indirect Coombs test (ICT) if negative at 12 weeks. Then at 12 weeks, repeat at 28th and 36th weeks in primi, in multigravidas—test if repeated at monthly intervals from 24th weeks onward, ICT +ve, referred to specialized fetal medicine unit (FMU) if repeat at 2 weeks to see for increasing titers.

FETAL MEDICINE UNIT REFERRAL

Rising antibody levels/titers or a level/titer above a specific threshold—anti-D levels >4 IU/mL, anti-C level of >7.5 IU/mL, any level of anti-K antibodies, anti-E potentiates the severity of fetal anemia due to anti-C antibodies so that referral at lower levels/titers is indicated; ultrasound suggestive of fetal anemia, a history of unexplained severe neonatal jaundice or neonatal anemia requiring transfusion or exchange transfusion, for antibodies other than anti-D, anti-C and anti-K—a history of previous significant hemolytic disease of the fetus and newborn (HDFN) or intrauterine transfusion (IUT), or a titer of 32 or above, especially if the titer is rising as rising titers correlate with increasing risk and severity of anemia.

Quantitative estimation of IgG antibody at weekly intervals, sudden rise in titer from 1:8 to 1:256 suggestive of fetal affection/1:16 titer/Ab level > 10 IU/mL → critical value → amniotic fluid optical density at 450 nm (OD450) and weekly USG to detect fetal hydrops. Doppler USG → peak flow velocity in middle cerebral artery (MCA) >1.5 multiples of the median (MoM) for that corresponding gestational age → moderate/severe fetal anemia. Amniocentesis and estimation of bilirubin in amniotic fluid by spectrophotometry → plotting in Liley's zone. **Figure 1** shows Liley's chart and **Figure 2** shows its Queenan chart modification.

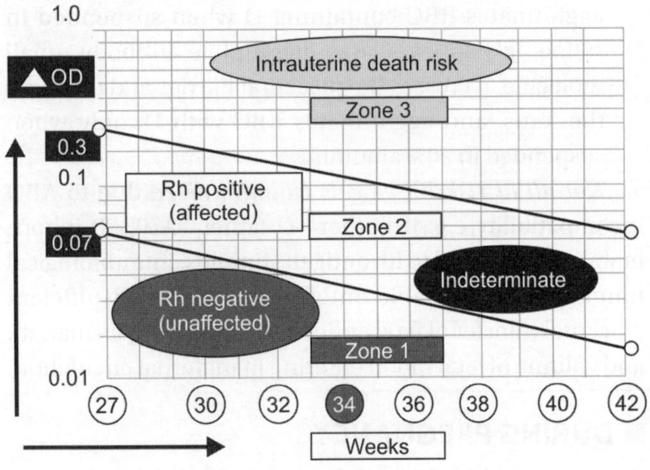

Fig. 1: Liley's chart.

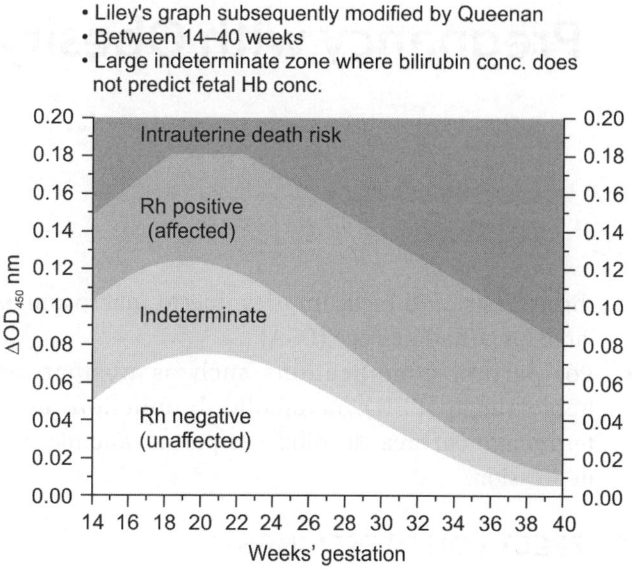

Fig. 2: Queenan's chart.

Prediction–Liley's Zone 1 (Low Zone)

Fetus unlikely to be affected, pregnancy continued to term; *Liley's zone 2 (mid zone)*—repeat at 2 weeks, if value ups → cordocentesis → Hct <30% → IUT to ↑ 40–45%, preterm delivery >34 weeks. *Liley's zone 3 (high zone)*—fetus severely affected and imminent death. Pregnancy >34 weeks—termination; <34 weeks → cordocentesis → Hct <30% → IUT ↑ Hct 40–45%. Preterm delivery >34 weeks.

- *Advantages:* Predict degree of hemolysis accurately, assessment of fetal anemia more accurate by cordocentesis
- *Plan of delivery:* **Unimmunized** mothers—expectant attitude, EDD should not overrun, **immunized** mothers—specialized centers with neonatal intensive care unit (NICU), facilities for exchange transfusion, expert neonatologist, mild affection → termination at 38 weeks of pregnancy, severe affection → terminate pregnancy at 34 weeks after steroid coverage and till then intrauterine fetal transfusion (intraperitoneal/intravascular) to continue pregnancy to 34 weeks.
- *Mode of delivery:* Induction of labor (IOL) with prostaglandins followed by ARM +/- Oxytocin; LSCS in premature termination with poor Bishop score and considering the severity of affection and urgency of termination
- *Care during delivery:* Vaginal delivery → continuous fetal monitoring to detect fetal distress, no Ergometrine, gentle handling of uterus in third stage, and care of PPH. LSCS—avoid spillage of blood in peritoneal cavity, routine MRP should be withheld:
    - Cord blood collection
    - Clotted blood—ABO and Rh typing, direct Coombs test (DCT), and serum bilirubin
    - Oxalated blood—hemoglobin, blood smear for immature RBC.

INTRAUTERINE FETAL TRANSFUSION

Severely affected fetus <34 weeks; advantages—correction of fetal anemia and improvement of oxygenation, improved fetal hepatic function. Methods—intraperitoneal → O-ve (Hct 80%) = gestational weeks—20 × 10 mL, intravascular → umbilical cord vein near its insertion into placenta.

Other therapies—plasmapheresis, high-dose IV immunoglobulin, etc. to mother and neonatal exchange transfusion, adjuvant therapy—photo therapy, photochemical therapy, Phenobarbitone inhibiting hemolysis—high-dose intravenous immunoglobin.

SUGGESTED READING

1. NICE. (2023). Ectopic pregnancy and miscarriage: diagnosis and initial management NICE, guideline [NG126]. [online] Available from https://www.nice.org.uk/guidance/ng126 [Last accessed September, 2024].
2. Prevention of Rh D Alloimmunization ACOG Practice Bulletin, Number 181. Obstet Gynecol. 2017;130(2): e57-e70.
3. RCOG. (2014). The Management of Women with Red Cell Antibodies during Pregnancy (Green-top Guideline No. 65). [online] Available from https://www.rcog.org.uk/guidance/browse-all-guidance/green-top-guidelines/the-management-of-women-with-red-cell-antibodies-during-pregnancy-green-top-guideline-no-65/ [Last accessed September, 2024].

CHAPTER 12

Pregnancy with Obesity

INTRODUCTION

World Health Organization (WHO) categorizes body mass index (BMI) into six groups—(1) underweight <18.5 kg/m^2, (2) normal weight 18.5–24.9 kg/m^2, (3) overweight 25–29.9 kg/m^2, and (4) obesity class I 30–34.9 kg/m^2, (5) class II 35–39.9 kg/m^2, and (6) class III/Morbid obesity ≥40 kg/m^2.

PRECONCEPTION CARE

Counseling about risks associated and advise to decrease BMI by lifestyle interventions, behavioral interventions, and encourage physical activity—exercise and dietary modifications. If not effective then seek pharmacological treatment like Orlistat (BMI ≥30 kg/m^2/≥28 kg/m^2 with risk factors). Bariatric surgery to be offered after multidisciplinary team (MDT) discussion in cases with BMI ≥40 kg/m^2 or 35–39.9 kg/m^2 and comorbidities, with contraception and nutritional advice at least for 12–18 months. BMI ≥30 kg/m^2 trying for pregnancy should take 5 mg Folic acid daily, at least 1 month before conception and continue during the first trimester of pregnancy. Obese women are at high risk of vitamin D deficiency but the evidence on whether routine vitamin D should be given to improve maternal and offspring outcomes remains uncertain.

EFFECTS ON PREGNANCY

- ↑ Risk of spontaneous miscarriage and recurrent miscarriages, congenital anomalies like neural tube defect (NTD), spina bifida, hydrocephalus, cardiovascular, orofacial and limb reduction anomalies, stillbirth, macrosomia, and fetal growth restriction (FGR)
- ↑ Pregnancy-induced hypertension (PIH), pre-eclampsia (PE), gestational diabetes mellitus (GDM), venous thromboembolism (VTE), cardiac dysfunction, sleep apnea, and nonalcoholic fatty liver disease
- Intrapartum complications such as preterm labor, increased risk of cesarean delivery, failed trial of labor, endometritis, wound rupture or dehiscence, venous thrombosis, and birth injuries due to macrosomia/large for gestational age (LGA)
- Postpartum complications such as postpartum hemorrhage (PPH), metabolic dysfunction, early termination of breastfeeding, postpartum anemia, and depression.

EFFECTS ON OFFSPRINGS

Childhood obesity, metabolic syndrome, asthma, autistic spectrum disorders, childhood developmental delay, and attention-deficit/hyperactivity disorder.

For patients with prepregnancy BMI 35.0–39.9, weekly antenatal fetal surveillance from 37 weeks of gestation and for BMI ≥40, it should begin at 34 weeks of gestation as at high risk of stillborn.

Antenatal Care

High-risk pregnancy (HRP), booked in consultant-led clinic, moving and handling risk assessment, informed decision regarding risks, dietary modification to optimize weight gain during pregnancy (anti-obesity/weight loss drugs **not** recommended during pregnancy), screen for GDM, appropriate size cuff for BP (standard, 12 × 23 cm; large, 15 × 33 cm; and thigh, 18 × 36 cm), Folic acid 5 mg daily, 150 mg Aspirin daily from 12 weeks of gestation till delivery, VTE risk assessment and thromboprophylaxis accordingly, screen for mental health problems—depression and anxiety, screening for fetal aneuploidy—trisomy 21 (Down syndrome), 18 and 13 using first trimester combined screening [maternal age + double markers + nuchal translucency (NT)-nasal bone (NB) scan], noninvasive prenatal testing (NIPT) has high chance of failure, and second-trimester fetal anomaly scan between 18^{+0} and 20^{+6} weeks of gestation to detect structural abnormalities (with limitation), serial measurement of symphysis fundal height (SFH) at each antenatal visit from 24 weeks of gestation small for gestational age (SGA)/LGA and if inaccurate then alternative/complimentary USG for serial assessment of fetal size; in third-trimester obstetric anesthetist referral for risk assessment regarding venous access, and regional and general anesthesia, and tissue viability issues.

INTRAPARTUM CARE

Intrapartum fetal monitoring [continuous electronic fetal monitoring (CEFM) in high-risk cases with comorbidities], options of IOL (for macrosomia, etc.) versus lower section cesarean section (LSCS) should be discussed according to individual woman's comorbidities, antenatal complications, and wishes; active management of the third stage of labor (AMTSL) to reduce PPH, venous access established early in labor and siting of a second cannula can be considered, additional measures to prevent pressure sores, transverse infra-panniculus skin incisions in LSCS preferred, prophylactic antibiotics and >2 cm subcutaneous fat should be sutured to reduce the risk of wound infection and wound dehiscence. No evidence to recommend routine use of negative pressure dressing, barrier retractors, and subcutaneous drains to reduce the risk of wound infection.

POSTPARTUM CARE

Breastfeeding support, venous thromboembolism (VTE) thromboprophylaxis along with early mobilization, and avoid dehydration; adequate follow-up for PIH/GDM; supported for weight loss and postnatal contraception (IUCD best, avoid hormonal). Behavioral counseling to improve healthy diet and exercise in order to achieve a healthier weight before another pregnancy.

SUGGESTED READING

1. Denison FC, Aedla NR, Keag O, Hor K, Reynolds RM, Milne A, et al. (2018). Care of Women with Obesity in Pregnancy (Green-top Guideline No. 72). BJOG. 2019;126(3): e62-e106.
2. National Institute for Health and Care Excellence (NICE). Obesity: identification, assessment and management Clinical guideline (CG) 189. [online] Available from https://nice.org.uk/guidance/cg189 [Last accessed September, 2024].
3. Obesity in Pregnancy ACOG Practice Bulletin, Number 230. Obstet Gynecol. 2021;137(6):e128-e144.

CHAPTER 13

Very Advanced Maternal Age

DEFINITION

Advanced maternal age is defined as women who are ≥35 years at estimated date of delivery, and "very advanced maternal age" (VAMA) refer to women who are aged ≥45 years at the time of delivery. Women aged ≥35 years are at higher risk for complications such as gestational diabetes, preeclampsia, labor dystocia, and cesarean delivery. Also, at risk of delivering a neonate who is born preterm (spontaneous or iatrogenic), increase low birth weight (LBW), low 5-minute Apgar score, and neonatal intensive care unit (NICU) admission.

FASTER (first- and second-trimester evaluation of risk) trial has demonstrated a significant association between chromosomal abnormalities and congenital malformations in offsprings of women aged ≥35 years.

ROLE OF ARTIFICIAL REPRODUCTIVE TECHNIQUES

Approximately three-fourths of women conceived >45 years by artificial reproductive techniques (ART), using donor gametes/embryo. ART itself associated with complications—ovarian hyperstimulation syndrome (OHSS), miscarriage, ectopic, pregnancy-induced hypertension (PIH), preeclampsia (PE), venous thromboembolism (VTE), genetic/chromosomal and structural malformations of fetus, fetal growth restriction (FGR), LBW, stillborn, and preterm labor—spontaneous/induced. These further increase with maternal age and multiple pregnancy.

RISKS OF VERY ADVANCED MATERNAL AGE: MATERNAL RISKS

- Early pregnancy complications such as miscarriage (~50%), ectopic pregnancy (↑X3 times) requiring BT
- Multiple pregnancy (due to double embryo transfer in ART) and its associated risks like antepartum hemorrhage (APH), PIH, gestational diabetes mellitus (GDM), ↑need of lower segment cesarean section (LSCS) and intensive care unit (ICU) admission
- Medical comorbidities—GDM, gestational hypertension, preeclampsia, hypothyroidism, and VTE
- Obstetric complications—placenta previa causing APH, placenta accreta spectrum (PAS) (especially if previous uterine surgery), PPH requiring BT, ↑cesarean delivery and prolonged hospital stay
- ↑ BMI and its associated risks
- ↑ ICU admission due to cardiac morbidity, renal failure, shock, and severe complications of obstetric interventions.

Fetal risks—↑ preterm births, LBW, small for gestational age (SGA), fetal growth restriction (FGR), ↓-APGAR and ↑ NICU admission, stillborn or neonatal demise, trisomy 21 (Down syndrome), and other chromosomal and congenital anomalies.

MANAGEMENT

- Prepregnancy counseling—risks associated with, both maternal and fetal condition explained
- High-risk pregnancy (HRP), booked in consultant-led clinic, MDT (maternal medicine/high-risk obs/multiple pregnancy clinic)
- Personalized care plan, ↓ BMI in obesity, and single embryo transfer in ART
- Folic acid (FA) 400 μg [5 mg in obesity, preexisting diabetes, and medical condition like sickle cell disease (SCD)/thalassemia, on medications like antiepileptics]
- Review medications if on antihypertensives, ECHO, renal function test (RFT), and renal imaging
- VTE risk assessment in each visit
- Early pregnancy—rule out miscarriage, ectopic, and multiple pregnancy
- Booking appointment—complete history regarding method of conception, any previous uterine surgery, booking scan for dating, FA (400 μg/5 mg if risk factor), low-dose Aspirin (LDA) (150 mg from 12 weeks till delivery)

- Individualized ANC in HRP clinic—pregnancy-associated plasma protein-A (PAPP-A) measured (sig. <0.4 MoM), serial growth scan at 28, 32, and 36 weeks, umbilical artery Doppler from 26 to 28 weeks of gestation (↑ risk of SGA/LGA)
- Fetal surveillance—aneuploidy screening by level-I NT-NB scan, combined test (with Double markers), noninvasive prenatal testing (NIPT) and if positive then confirmatory invasive tests—CVS/amniocentesis for any genetic/chromosomal abnormalities; level-II anomaly scan at 18–20 weeks to rule out structural anomalies (cardiac defects)
- Screen for GDM at 16–18 weeks, and if negative repeat at 26–28 weeks
- Regular blood pressure monitoring and urine tests (rule out preeclampsia), treat anemia
- Maternal medicine, obstetric anesthetic referral if ↑ BMI, HTN, GDM, and multiple pregnancy
- Counseling regarding risk of preterm delivery, mode, and place of delivery with NICU facility
- Deliver by induction of labor at 39 weeks to ↓ risk of stillborn. LSCS only for obstetric indications not done for advanced age. PPH prophylaxis by uterotonics.

SUGGESTED READING

1. American College of Obstetricians and Gynecologists' Committee on Clinical Consensus-Obstetrics; Gantt A; Society for Maternal-Fetal Medicine; Metz TD, Kuller JA, Louis JM; Cahill AG, Turrentine M. Obstetric Care Consensus #11, Pregnancy at age 35 years or older. Am J Obstet Gynecol. 2023;228(3):B25-B40.
2. Howell A, Blott M. Very advanced maternal age. Obstetr Gynaecol. 2021;23:38-47.

CHAPTER 14

Teenage Pregnancy

DEFINITION

When pregnancy occurs before age of 20 years (between 13 and 19 years).

RISK FACTORS

Socioeconomic deprivation, low educational achievement, those in care of social services, mental health problems, domestic violence, sexual abuse, crime, or rape.

IMPACT/OUTCOME OF TEENAGE PREGNANCY—MATERNAL

- Antepartum—eclampsia, anemia, pregnancy-induced hypertension (PIH), preeclampsia, miscarriage, and preterm labor (<32 weeks)
- Intrapartum—prolonged labor, obstructed labor, and ↑ chance of instrumental deliveries, systemic infections
- Postpartum—postpartum hemorrhage (PPH), postnatal depression, or blues, puerperal endometritis.

Fetal Outcome

Low birth weight (LBW), preterm birth, small for gestational age (SGA), fetal growth restriction (FGR), ↑neonatal morbidity and mortality.

Offspring Outcome

- Poor cognitive development, low education attainment, ↑risk of abuse, neglect and behavioral problem, and ↑criminal activity
- Cause of poor fetomaternal outcome is gynecological immaturity and poor maternal growth and nutrition leading to FGR (competition for nutrients between maternal body and gravid uterus).

RISKS ASSOCIATED WITH TEENAGE PREGNANCY

- Poor diet due to poor eating habits and neglect vitamins, there is poor weight gain in pregnancy leading to LBW babies.
- *Sexually transmitted infection (STI):* There is increased association with sexually transmitted diseases (may lead to ectopic pregnancy) and its complications.
- Illicit drug or substance abuse, alcohol and smoking may lead to abruptio, preterm premature rupture of the fetal membrane (PPROM), preterm birth, stillbirth, and sudden infant death syndrome (SIDS). Even passive exposure to smoke is a risk factor for respiratory infection, asthma, allergy, and adverse neurodevelopmental of child.
- Postnatal depression and difficulties with breastfeeding due to decreased milk production along with differences in breastfeeding behavior need extrasupport.

MANAGEMENT

- General—supportive care, social support in a non-judgmental manner
- Medical termination of pregnancy (MTP) due to unplanned and unwanted pregnancy, they may seek unskilled practices and/or dangerous methods leading to life-threatening complications.
- After pregnancy termination, suitable contraception ("Double Dutch") to prevent unwanted pregnancy as well as STI [Barrier + other effective method (COC/Implant)]
- *ANC:* If willing to continue pregnancy, it will be considered as high-risk pregnancy (HRP), booked at consultant led clinic, confirm gestational age (GA), booking scan, and antenatal advice—nutritious diet, supplement vitamins, and stop any addiction with input from social services
- IPC due to immature bony pelvis, ↑chance of prolonged, and obstructed labor so strict vigilance during active labor
- *PNC:* Counseling and education regarding infant feeding, growth, and safety need because of ↑risk of infant dying in first year of life.
- Contraception, sexual education, financial issues, and pursue school/college education.

SUGGESTED READING

1. WHO: Fact sheets on Adolescent Pregnancy.

NOTES

NOTES

SECTION 3

Labor Disorders

Section Authors: *Shashi Bala Arya, Preeti Singh, Anuradha Sharma, Sunaina Chandra*

CHAPTER 15

Cephalopelvic Disproportion

INTRODUCTION

Labor refers to the presence of uterine contractions of sufficient intensity, frequency, and duration to bring about demonstrable effacement and dilation of the cervix. Abnormal labor results from abnormalities of the power, passenger, and passage (pelvis or soft tissues). The term "cephalopelvic disproportion (CPD)" means disparity between the size of the maternal pelvis and the fetal head that precludes vaginal delivery. Obstructed labor is a common complication of undiagnosed CPD in labor.

Cesarean birth indicated by CPD accounts for a significant increase in cesarean section rate (CSR). According to World Health Organization (WHO) recommendations, the optimal CSR due to CPD should not be >5%.

TYPES

- *Absolute CPD* is true mechanical obstruction resulting from contracted pelvis, pelvic exostoses, spondylolisthesis, and anterior sacrococcygeal tumors. Some temporary fetal contributions are hydrocephalus and macrosomia.
- *Relative CPD* resulting from malpresentation and malposition such as brow presentation, face presentation, mentoposterior, and occipitoposterior positions.

DIAGNOSIS

Diagnosis of CPD is difficult as we know that fetal head is best pelvimeter, barring cases of absolute CPD, relative CPD can only be suspected and screened before labor, only to be confirmed in labor.

Suspicion of CPD to be raised in women with history of previous difficult deliveries, abnormalities in her height, weight, gait, delay in engagement, and shape of abdomen (pendulous). Clinical features of dystocia dystrophia syndrome include obese stocky built women with broad shoulders and short thighs.

SCREENING TOOLS

- Abdominal method
- Abdominopelvic method
- External pelvimetry
- Internal pelvimetry
- Radiological methods (not in practice now)

Abdominal Method (Fig. 1)

Patient placed in recumbent dorsal position with thigh flexed and slightly abducted. Fetal head is grasped by left hand. Two fingers (index and middle) of the right hand are placed above the symphysis pubis keeping inner surface of fingers in line with the symphysis pubis to note the degree of overlapping if any when the head is pushed downward and backward.

Abdominopelvic Method (Muller–Munro-Kerr Method) (Fig. 2)

- External hand pushes the head into the pelvis, while fingers of the other (internal) hand estimates the relative size of pelvis and head. Thumb of internal

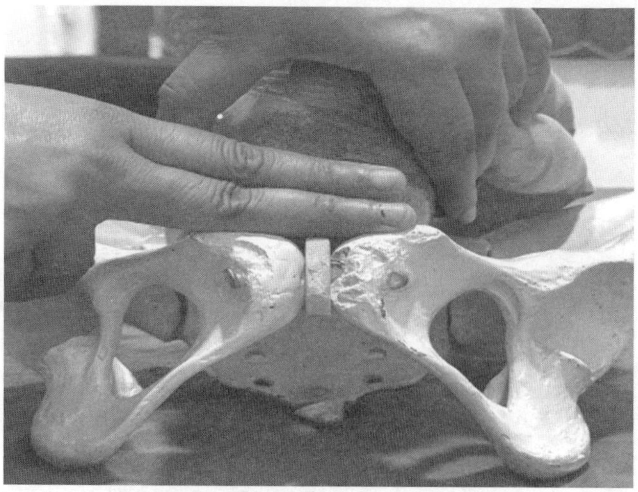

Fig. 1: Abdominal method of cephalopelvic disproportion (CPD) assessment.

hand is externally palpating the pubic symphysis and its relative position with fetal head.

- *Interpretation:*
  - *No disproportion:* Head can be pushed till ischial spine.
  - *Moderate disproportion:* Parietal bones flush with symphysis pubis.
  - *Severe disproportion:* Parietal bones overhanging on and hitting the thumb or index finger resting on symphysis pubis.

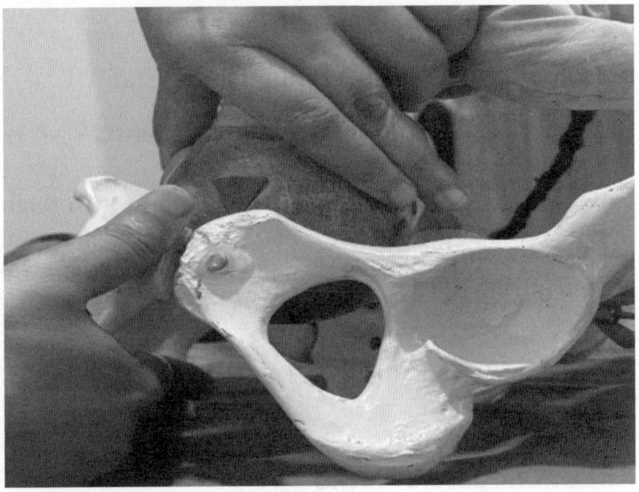

Fig. 2: Abdominopelvic method of cephalopelvic disproportion (CPD) assessment.

External Pelvimetry (Figs. 3A to C)

Tools required:

- Collins pelvimeter
- Foot gauge
- *Stadiometer:*
  - Interspinous diameter (25 cm) between anterior superior iliac spines (ASIS)
  - Intercrestal diameter (28 cm) between two farthest points over iliac crest
  - External conjugate (20 cm) midpoint of symphysis pubis and lower border of L5 vertebra
  - Foot length (23 cm) the distance from acropodion (it is the most forwardly projecting point on the tip of the first or second toe whichever is longer, when the person stands erect) to pternion (it is the most backwardly projecting point on the heel, when the person stands upright with equal pressure on both feet)
  - Maternal standing height (145 cm)

Internal Pelvimetry

Assess at all three levels of pelvis: Inlet, cavity and outlet.

- Detects diminished diameters of pelvis.
- Provides an idea about the overall shape and type of the pelvis.
- Though subjective but with practice finding can be made reproducible.

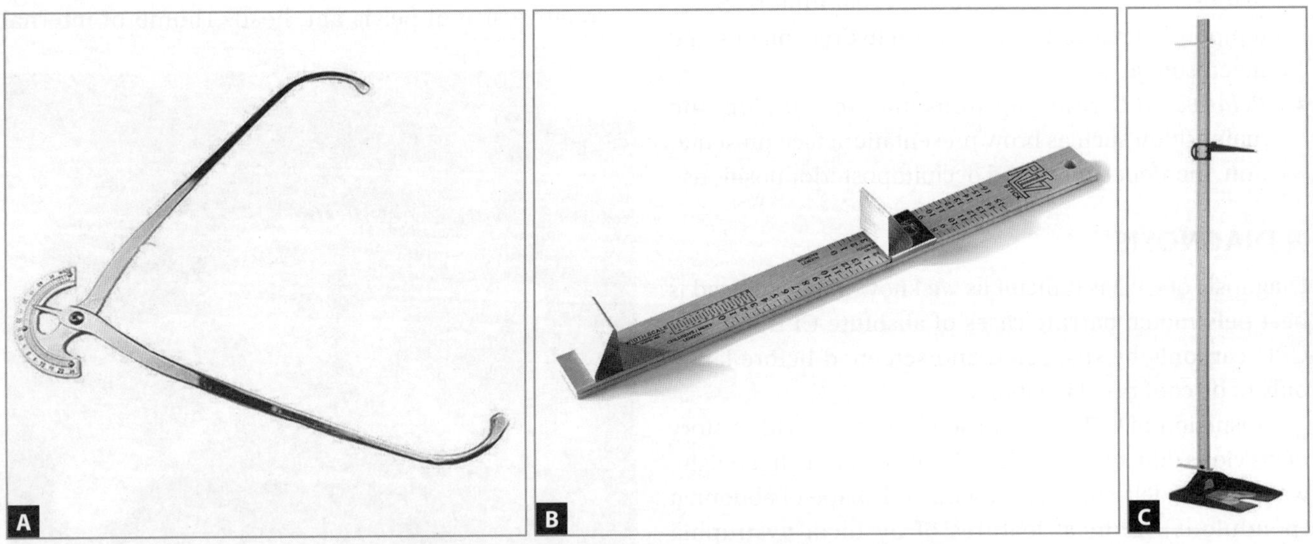

Figs. 3A to C: (A) Collin's pelvimeter; (B) Foot gauge; (C) Stadiometer.

- Midpelvis [interspinous distance (ISD) <8–10 cm] assessment is difficult.
- Idea about midpelvis can be drawn by transverse diameter of outlet (TDO) <10 cm.
- Sacrum should be smooth, short, and well curved. Straight and long sacrum is abnormal.
- Sacrosciatic notch sufficient wide to accommodate two fingers, tells about the posterior segment of pelvis and side walls of lower pelvis
- Ischial spine—smooth and everted not prominent and not felt into the pelvis
- Sidewalls—parallel
- Posterior surface of pubic symphysis—smooth
- Sacro coccygeal joint mobility and state of coccyx
- Configuration of pubic arch; round and two finger width
- Subpubic angle corresponds to the fully abducted thumb and index finger, acute is abnormal.
- TDO <10 cm, four knuckles width
- Anteroposterior (AP) diameter of the outlet can be measured by an external caliper distance between inferior margin of pubic symphysis to sacrococcygeal joint.

CEPHALOPELVIC DISPROPORTION IN LABOR IF FOLLOWING FEATURES ARE OBSERVED

- Large fetal size
- Fetal head overriding the pubic symphysis
- Cervix shrinking after amniotomy
- Edema of the cervix
- Head not well applied against the cervix
- Head not engaged with leading point at -2 station
- Caput formation
- Moulding (cranial bones overlapping)
- Deflexion (anterior fontanelle easily palpable)
- Asynclitism (sagittal suture is not in the middle of the pelvis).

MANAGEMENT OPTIONS

- Trial of labor—conduction of spontaneous labor in mild-to-moderate degree of CPD at inlet and cavity in an institution under supervision with watchful expectancy aiming at vaginal delivery
- Cesarean delivery

  Indications are:
  - Moderate-to-severe disproportion with obstetric complication
  - Obstetric conjugate is <7.5 cm
  - Contracted outlet
  - Moderate contracted midpelvis associated with outlet abnormality
  - Severely contracted midpelvis

Guidelines were revised by Society for Maternal-Fetal Medicine (SMFM) and American College of Obstetricians and Gynecologists (ACOG) 2014 and recommendations to diagnose abnormal progress of labor (due to CPD) are as follows:

- Active phase defined by cervical dilatation of at least 6 cm together with no cervical change in spite of adequate uterine activity for at least 4 hours (or at least 6 hours of Oxytocin administration with inadequate uterine activity)
- Arrest of labor in the second stage of labor for at least 2 or 3 hours respectively of pushing in multiparous or nulliparous women
- Prelabor cesarean delivery to avoid potential birth trauma in cases of estimated fetal weights of at least 5,000 g in women without diabetes and at least 4,500 g in women with diabetes.

SUGGESTED READING

1. Baskett TF, Calder AA, Arulkumaran S. Munro Kerr's Operative Obstetrics, 13th edition. Philadelphia: Elsevier Saunders; 2020.
2. Cunningham F, Leveno KJ, Dashe JS, Hoffman BL, Spong CY, Casey BM. Williams Obstetrics, 26th edition. Philadelphia: McGraw Hill; 2022.
3. Symonds I, Arulkumaran S. Essentials of Obstetrics, 5th edition. Philadelphia: Churchill Livingstone Publishers Pvt. Limited; 2013.

CHAPTER 16

Preterm Labor

DEFINITION

Preterm labor is defined as onset of labor before 37th completed weeks but after the period of viability, i.e., 28 weeks of gestation, in developing countries (24 weeks in developed countries). According to recent NICE guideline:

- ***Established*** *preterm labor:* If progressive cervical dilatation ≥4 cm with regular uterine contractions, i.e., active preterm labor.
- ***Suspected*** *preterm labor:* If symptoms of preterm labor + on P/S or P/V confirm preterm labor, but rule out established labor, i.e., <4 cm cervical dilatation.
- ***Diagnosed*** *preterm labor:* If she is in suspected, i.e., symptoms and signs of preterm labor + positive diagnostic test for preterm labor.

INCIDENCE

About 5–10%.

RISK FACTORS

- Demographic factors—race (black >>), low body mass index (BMI), poor maternal weight gain, age <17 years/>35 years, poor education, women living alone, minimal/no prenatal care, low socioeconomic status, and ↑ number of partners
- Psychosocial factors—anxiety, stress, depression, negative life events, racial discrimination, domestic violence, working >42 hours a week/>6 hours a day, work-stress/dissatisfaction, and smoking
- Past obstetric history—preterm birth/midtrimester loss, >3 first trimester abortions
- Pregnancy following assisted reproductive techniques.

CAUSES

Multifactorial:

- Maternal—pregnancy complications— preeclampsia, antepartum hemorrhage, and premature rupture of membrane (PE, APH, and PROM)
    - Overdistension of uterus—multiple pregnancy, polyhydramnios, and large for gestational age (LGA) baby
    - Uterine abnormalities—cervical incompetence and congenital uterine anomalies
    - Medical/surgical—fever, recurrent urinary tract infection (UTI), pyelonephritis, appendicitis, diarrhea, etc.
    - Chronic disease—hypertension (HTN), diabetes mellitus (DM), chronic renal disease, heart disease, etc.
    - Genital tract infections—BV, *Bacteroides*, Chlamydia, *Mycoplasma*
- Fetal—multiple pregnancy congenital malformation, intrauterine device (IUD)
- Placental—infarction, thrombosis, abruptio, and previa
- Iatrogenic—medical/obstetric complications
- Idiopathic

Flowchart 1 depicts the etiopathogenesis of preterm labor.

Flowchart 1: Etiopathogenesis of preterm labor.

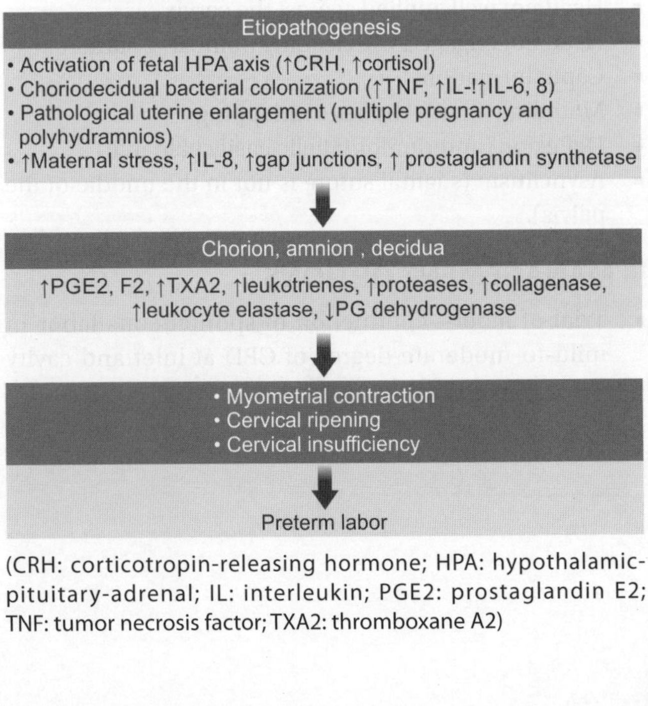

(CRH: corticotropin-releasing hormone; HPA: hypothalamic-pituitary-adrenal; IL: interleukin; PGE2: prostaglandin E2; TNF: tumor necrosis factor; TXA2: thromboxane A2)

DIAGNOSIS

- Symptoms—pelvic pressure, backache, and discharge/bleeding per vaginum (PV)
- Signs—regular uterine contractions 4 in 20 minutes/8 in 60 minutes (lasting ≥40 seconds), cervical changes—dilatation >1 cm and effacement >80%, length of cervix <1.5 cm and funneling of internal os.

PREDICTORS OF PRETERM LABOR

- *Clinical:* History of abortion/preterm birth, asymptomatic bacteriuria/recurrent UTI, genital tract infection, multiple pregnancy/polyhydramnios.
- *Biophysical:* Uterine contractions, cervical length <2.5 cm, funneling (int. os >5 mm), bishop score >4, serial transvaginal sonography (TVS) for cervical length beginning at 16 weeks of gestation and repeated until 24 weeks for individuals with singleton pregnancy and prior spontaneous preterm birth is recommended.
- *Biochemical:* Fetal fibronectin (extracellular glycoprotein secreted by chorionic tissue) in cervicovaginal discharge at 24–37 weeks >50 ng/mL, IL-6 and 8, and tumor necrosis factor alpha (TNF-α).

MANAGEMENT

Aims

- To prevent onset of preterm labor
- To arrest the preterm labor
- Appropriate management of labor
- Effective neonatal care

Investigations

- Complete blood count, blood glucose, urine routine analysis, culture and sensitivity, high vaginal swab culture, and vaginal fibronectin
- Ultrasonography for fetal wellbeing, effective fetal weight, amniotic fluid, and placental localization.

Measures to Prevent Preterm Labor

- To reduce incidence of preterm labor by appropriate management of risk factors such as infection and smoking
- Screening tests for early detection
- Prophylactic management (cerclage/tocolysis)

Measures to Arrest Preterm Labor

If fetus not compromised, maternal condition good, no PROM—bed rest, adequate hydration, prophylactic antibiotic treatment (if infective etiology), tocolysis, neuroprotection, and corticosteroid administration.

- *Role of tocolysis in preterm labor:* Short-term therapy (recommended from 26 to <34 weeks), mainly for two indications—(1) steroid coverage and (2) in utero transfer to center with neonatal intensive care unit (NICU); Nifedipine is the drug of choice, if contraindicated, Atosiban is preferred. Use of betamimetics is not recommended.
- *Role of prophylactic vaginal progesterone or cervical cerclage:* If cervical length <25 mm between 16 and 24 weeks of gestation + history of spontaneous preterm birth (up to 34 weeks of gestations) or midtrimester loss (after 16 weeks of gestation). **Only vaginal PGN** till 34 weeks, if positive history **or** TVS suggestive of cervical length <2.5 cm. **Prophylactic cervical cerclage**, if TVS suggestive of cervix <2.5 cm and either PT PROM in previous pregnancy or cervical trauma [cone biopsy/large loop excision of the transformation zone (LLETZ)].
- *Maternal corticosteroids:* It is recommended from 24 to 34^{+6} weeks and can be considered from 34^{+6} to <36 weeks if suspected/diagnosed/established preterm labor. For planned cesarean between 37^{+0} and 38^{+6} weeks an informed decision-making with respect to benefits (↓NICU admission due to respiratory morbidity). versus risks (hypoglycemia and developmental delay).
- *Role of neuroprotection in preterm labor:* Intravenous Magnesium Sulfate is recommended between 24 and 29^{+6} weeks and considered from 30 to 33^{+6} weeks who are in established preterm labor or having a planned preterm birth within 24 hours. *Dose recommended:* 4 g (20%) intravenous bolus Magnesium sulfate over 15 minutes, followed by an intravenous infusion of 1 g per hour until the birth or for 24 hours (whichever is sooner). Monitor for clinical signs of Magnesium toxicity at least every 4 hours by recording pulse, blood pressure, respiratory rate, and deep tendon reflexes.

Management in Labor

- *Aim:* Prevent birth asphyxia and respiratory distress syndrome (RDS), birth trauma, and ensure NICU facility

- *First stage:*
  - Patient is put to bed to prevent early rupture of membranes, hydration, and sedation
  - Careful labor monitoring with continuous electronic fetal heart monitoring
  - Epidural analgesia is of choice.
  - No fetal blood sampling (FBS)/fetal scalp electrodes (FSE)
  - Cesarean delivery is done for obstetric reasons only.
  - Consider cesarean birth for women presenting in suspected, diagnosed or established preterm labor between 26^{+0} and 36^{+6} weeks of pregnancy with breech presentation.
- *Second stage:*
  - Birth should be slow and gentle to avoid rapid compression and decompression of head.
  - Liberal episiotomy should be given to minimize head compression.
  - Forceps if tendency to delay, no ventouse <34 weeks
  - Cord clamping can be delayed for up to 60 seconds, unless contraindicated.
  - Position the baby at or below the level of the placenta before clamping the cord
  - Baby should be shifted to NICU under neonatologist.
- *Care of a preterm neonate:*
  - Cord to be kept long 10–12 cm.
  - Air passage should be cleared of mucus promptly.
  - Adequate oxygenation (concentration <35%)
  - Wrap baby including head in sterile warm towel to prevent hypothermia
  - Aqueous solution of vitamin K
  - Intensive care protocols

SUGGESTED READING

1. NICE. (2022). Preterm labour and birth NICE guideline [NG25]. [online] Available from https://www.nice.org.uk/guidance/ng25 [Last accessed September, 2024].
2. Prediction and Prevention of Spontaneous Preterm Birth ACOG Practice Bulletin Number 234. Obstet Gynecol. 2021; 138(2):e65-e90.
3. Stock SJ, Thomson AJ, Papworth S; Royal College of Obstetricians and Gynaecologists. Antenatal corticosteroids to reduce neonatal morbidity and mortality. Green-top Guideline No. 74. BJOG. 2022;129(8):e35-e60.

CHAPTER 17

Preterm Premature Rupture of Membranes

DEFINITION

Spontaneous rupture of fetal membranes before 37 completed weeks and before onset of labor. Associated with significant neonatal morbidity and mortality due to prematurity, sepsis, cord prolapse, pulmonary hypoplasia, neurodevelopmental impairment, chorioamnionitis, and abruptio.

INCIDENCE

3%, associated with 30–40% preterm births [Term prelabor rupture of membrane (PROM)—8%].

CAUSE

Intra-amniotic infection and oxidative stress-induced damage.

RISK FACTORS

- Low-socioeconomic status, body mass index (BMI) <19.8, nutritional deficiency, preterm prelabor rupture of membrane (PPROM) in previous pregnancy, multifetal gestation, and periodontal disease—gum inflammation are risk factors.
- *Pregnancy factor:* Threaten miscarriage in early pregnancy, fetal congenital defects. Interval between pregnancies <18 months or >59 months. Previous one preterm birth → ↑threefold risk.
- *Lifestyle factor:* Cigarette smoking, inadequate maternal weight gain, obese women, very young or aged mother, short stature, vitamins deficiency, depression, anxiety disorder, domestic violence, working long hours, and hard physical labor.
- *Genetic factor:* Familial and racial nature. Infection, bacterial vaginosis, associated with PPROM.

DIAGNOSIS

By typical maternal history followed by a sterile speculum examination shows draining liquor as pool of fluid (no further diagnostic test required). If, on P/S no amniotic fluid is observed then perform an insulin-like growth factor binding protein-1 (IGFBP-1) test or placental alpha-microglobulin-1 (PAMG-1) test of vaginal fluid for further management (No role of USG). Digital examination should be avoided unless the patient appears to be in active labor or delivery seems imminent, due to of introducing infection.

Symptoms of clinical chorioamnionitis—lower abdominal pain, abnormal vaginal discharge, fever, malaise, and reduced fetal movements. Combination of clinical features—pulse, blood pressure (BP), respiratory rate (RR), and temperature; blood tests [C-reactive protein and white blood cell (CRP and WBC)] and fetal heart rate [nonstress test (NST)] should be used to diagnose chorioamnionitis in women with PPROM.

MANAGEMENT

Outpatient management of PPROM with a viable fetus not recommended, so admit for evaluation. Periviable PROM may be considered for home care after a period of assessment in the hospital.

- *Erythromycin:* 250 mg four times a day for 10 days, or until the woman is in established labor (whichever is sooner), reduces chorioamnionitis, prolongs latency, and improves neonatal outcomes. Penicillin can be used who cannot tolerate Erythromycin, but Co-Amoxiclav should be avoided as it is associated with ↑risk of neonatal necrotizing enterocolitis.
- Corticosteroids (Betnesol/Dexona) from 24^{+0} till 35^{+6} weeks (ACOG-36^{+6} weeks) reduce the risks of respiratory distress syndrome and intraventricular hemorrhage.
- *Magnesium sulfate:* If in established labor or having a planned preterm birth within 24 hours, between 24^{+0} and 29^{+6} weeks (ACOG-32 weeks), ↓cerebral palsy and motor dysfunction in the offspring. Dose 4 g (20%) IV bolus $MgSO_4$ over 15 minutes, followed by IV infusion of 1 g/h until the birth or for 24 hours (whichever is sooner). Monitor for clinical signs of Mg toxicity

by 4-hourly—pulse, BP, RR, urine output, and deep tendon (patellar) reflexes. If develops oliguria or other evidence of renal failure reduce/stop $MgSO_4$.

- Emotional support during pregnancy and postpartum to ↓ post-traumatic stress disorder (PTSD)

Tocolysis and amnioinfusion are **not** recommended in PPROM.

TIMING OF BIRTH

If PPROM >24^{+0} weeks and *no contraindications* to continue the pregnancy, offer expectant management until 34^{+0} weeks, as associated with better outcomes for the mother and baby, with no difference in neonatal sepsis or infection. **"Exclusion criteria"**: Active labor, chorioamnionitis, concerns about fetal wellbeing, monochorionic multiple pregnancy, hypertensive disorders, etc. Expectant management—till no sign of chorioamnionitis/maternal or fetal compromise.

Either expectant management or immediate delivery from 34 weeks to 36^{+6} weeks balancing risk-benefit ratio. If any maternal/fetal compromise, induction of labor (IOL) done, lower segment cesarean section (LSCS) only for obstetric indications.

During preterm labor fetal blood sampling (FBS) and fetal scalp electrodes (FSE), ventouse contraindicated <34 weeks. *Group B Streptococcus* (GBS) prophylaxis only in labor. Timing of cord clamping for preterm babies (born vaginally or by cesarean birth)—at least 60 seconds before clamping the cord unless maternal or fetal conditions need earlier clamping. Position the baby at or below the level of the placenta before clamping the cord.

- ≥37 weeks—IOL, group B streptococcal prophylaxis recommended
- <24 weeks—Expectant management or IOL. Group B streptococcal prophylaxis not recommended; Corticosteroids are not recommended. Antimicrobials—there are incomplete data on use in prolonging latency, the combination of birthweight, gestational age, and sex provides the best estimate of chances of survival.

American College of Obstetricians and Gynecologists' recommends Ampicillin 2 g IV stat then 500 mg IV 6 hourly followed by Erythromycin 500 mg 6 hourly oral for next 10 day or till delivery which is sooner.

Next pregnancy: Risk of PPROM is increased. Progesterone is recommended in singleton pregnancy with history of prior spontaneous preterm birth (due to labor with intact membranes or preterm PROM).

SUGGESTED READING

1. NICE. (2015). Preterm labour and birth NICE guideline [NG25]. [online] Available from https://www.nice.org.uk/guidance/ng25 [Last accessed September, 2024].
2. Prelabor Rupture of Membranes ACOG Practice Bulletin PB Number 217. Obstet Gynecol. 2020;135(3):e80-e97.
3. RCOG. (2019). Care of Women Presenting with Suspected Preterm Prelabour Rupture of Membranes from 24^{+0} Weeks of Gestation RCOG Green-top Guideline No. 73. [online] Available from https://www.rcog.org.uk/guidance/browse-all-guidance/green-top-guidelines/care-of-women-presenting-with-suspected-preterm-prelabour-rupture-of-membranes-from-24plus0-weeks-of-gestation-green-top-guideline-no-73/ [Last accessed September, 2024].

CHAPTER 18

Prolonged Pregnancy

INTRODUCTION

"Post-term" pregnancy, "postmaturity", "postdates", and "prolonged pregnancy". The American College of Obstetrician and Gynecologist (ACOG), the World Health Organization (WHO), and the International Federation of Gynecology and Obstetrics (FIGO) have defined prolonged pregnancy as pregnancy at 42 completed weeks of gestation [i.e., 294 days after last menstrual period (LMP) or more]. Since there is a gradual decline in placental vascularity and its function, a postdated pregnancy may culminate in fetal distress and occasionally fetal death.

EPIDEMIOLOGY

- Incidence 7–11%
- 4% >43 weeks
- Recurrence 50%

Postmaturity Syndrome

It is characterized by prolonged gestation, sometimes a large sized fetus and diminished placental capacity for exchange associated with cutaneous and nutritional changes in the newborn infant.

Pregnancy should not be permitted to go beyond term in conditions like:

- Gestational hypertension
- Preeclampsia and eclampsia
- Renal diseases associated with pregnancy
- Chronic hypertension associated with pregnancy
- Rh isoimmunization in pregnancy
- Diabetes mellitus
- Antepartum hemorrhage

Causes of Post-term Pregnancy

- Incorrect dates (most frequent cause)
- *Fetal congenital abnormalities:*
    - Anencephaly (without hydramnios)
    - Adrenal hypoplasia
- *Maternal factors:*
    - Primipara, age >40 years, and obesity
    - Previous post-term pregnancy
    - Family occurrence
- *Placental factors:*
    - Deficiency of placental sulfatase
    - Deficiency of placental corticotropin-releasing hormone (CRH)
- Past history
- Family history

DIAGNOSIS

Diagnosis is often difficult because of inaccuracy of the date of the last menstrual period (as most of our women do not remember their LMP). It is also not possible in cases of irregular periods, lactational amenorrhea preceding pregnancy, and postpill amenorrhea. The time of diagnosis of pregnancy by urine test is important. In these cases, the examination of size of the uterus are useful. The date of quickening also helps, but most accurate is the earliest first-trimester ultrasound examination. NICE advise ultrasound scan in early pregnancy to determine gestational age using—CRL from 10^{+0} weeks to 13^{+6} weeks; head circumference (HC) if CRL is >84 mm.

On examination:

- *General examination:* Weight-falling/stationary on serial examinations
- *Abdominal examination:*
    - Uterine size to assess the period of gestation
    - Girth of the abdomen—steady decline due to reduced amniotic fluid volume
    - Increased prominence of the fetal parts to palpation
- *Ultrasound abdomen:*
    - Assessment of gestational age
    - Fetal weight
    - Fetal maturity [by biparietal diameter (BPD), HC, abdominal circumference (AC), and femur length (FL)]

- Restriction of fetal growth
- A loss of fetal subcutaneous fat
- Amount of liquor (oligohydramnios, amniotic fluid index ≤5 cm)
- Placental localization and maturity (Grade 3)

- Rule out cephalopelvic disproportion.

Doppler ultrasound has **no** proven value, till date, in the surveillance of post-term fetuses.

COMPLICATION

During Pregnancy

- *Oligohydramnios*: Reduced amniotic fluid volume in the absence of ruptured membranes or fetal urinary abnormalities is due to poor placental function leading to less renal blood flow and less urine output. Oligohydramnios usually associated with growth-restricted fetus.
- Cord compression
- Macrosomia
- Placenta insufficiency (fetal hypoxia)
- Fetal distress

During Labor

- *Maternal:*
    - Labor dysfunction (e.g., incoordinate uterine action)
    - Obstetric trauma
    - Increase operative/instrumental delivery
    - Hemorrhage
- *Fetal:*
    - Macrosomia
    - Shoulder dystocia—greater risk of operative delivery
    - Decreased moulding capacity (because the skull bones are no longer pliable and soft)
    - Cord compression
    - Fetal asphyxia

FOLLOWING DELIVERY

- *Appearance of the neonate at birth:* The post-term newborn has a wrinkled and yellow greenish colored skin, which is peeling at places (due to loss of protective effect of vernix caseosa). The body is long and thin suggestive of wasting. The newborn is usually alert, has wide open eye. Skin wrinkles are accentuated (especially in palms and soles). Finger and toenails are long with an appearance of advanced maturity.
- Increased incidence of neonatal convulsions
- Severe meconium aspiration syndrome (due to oligohydramnios if the liquor is meconium stained, thick, and viscous)
- Atelectasis of lungs
- Hypoglycemia
- Polycythemia
- Hyperbilirubinemia
- Low Apgar score (<4 at 5 minutes)
- Abnormal neurological signs
- Sleep disorders
- Inadequate social competence during the first year of life

Due to the complications mentioned above neonatal intensive care unit (NICU) admissions may be needed.

MANAGEMENT

A pregnant lady who has completed 41 weeks of pregnancy, should be admitted in the hospital and put on fetal surveillance. Expected fetal weight is assessed, and any cephalopelvic disproportion ruled out.

The level of fetal fibronectin in cervical secretion (if possible), is measured (a level of 50 mg/mL is observed to correlate with spontaneous labor within 3 days).

The patient should be instructed to keep a daily fetal movement record.

In case of any abnormalities on cardiotocographic tracings or on postcontraction fetal heart auscultation, an immediate delivery is indicated (vaginal or abdominal).

It is necessary to initiate fetal surveillance at 41 weeks of pregnancy—nonstress test and an assessment of amniotic fluid volume.

Induction of labor (IOL) is carried out if the nonstress test is nonreactive and amniotic fluid volume is 5 cm or less. It should also be done in women complaining of decreased fetal movements.

Oxytocin stress test is performed. If abnormal, it is an indication for delivery.

Sweeping and stripping of the membranes can be performed along with prostaglandin gel [prostaglandin E2 (PGE2) dinoprostone gel] in the nondilated cervix.

With a favorable cervix, Oxytocin drip is started combined with amniotomy. Early artificial rupture of membranes (ARM) helps in detection of thick meconium, which is important.

If the baby is big, it is best to be delivered by cesarean section.

NICE guideline recommends that IOL should be offered to women between 41^{+0} and 42^{+0} weeks. The reason for IOL at this time is to reduce the risks of prolonged pregnancy namely perinatal death, which increases with increasing gestational age.

The rates of operative vaginal delivery appear to be increased with IOL.

The rates of cesarean section do not appear to increase with IOL.

NICE guideline advises that women who decline IOL should daily have fetal monitoring performed in the form of CTG and liquor volume at least twice weekly.

RECOMMENDATIONS

- *Clinical practice guidelines SOGC committee opinion:*
    - Women who reach 41–42 weeks of gestation (uncomplicated pregnancies) should be offered elective delivery.
    - Serial fetal surveillance should consist (as a minimum) of an ultrasound assessment of amniotic fluid volume twice weekly and other forms of monitoring may be added to this [biophysical profile (BPP), NST, and fetal movement count].
- *Practical management of prolonged pregnancy:* When the woman reaches 41 weeks, she should meet with a consultant obstetrician. Women have a right to be informed of the small increase in risk associated with continuing the pregnancy after 41 weeks.

SUGGESTED READING

1. American College of Obstetrics and Gynaecologists: Management of post-term pregnancy. Practice Bulletin PB no. 6, Oct 1997.
2. Ballantyne JW. The problem of the post-mature infant. J Obstet Gynaecol Br Emp. 1902;2:521.
3. Divon MY, Haglund B, Nisell H, Otterblad PO, Westgren M. Foetal and neonatal mortality in post-term pregnancy: the impact of gestational age and foetal growth restriction. Am J Obstet Gynaecol. 1998;178:726.

CHAPTER 19

Breech

INCIDENCE

About 3–5% singleton pregnancies at term.

CLASSIFICATION

- Frank—legs extended
- Complete—all flexion
- Incomplete—1 hip extended
- Star gazing—hyperextended neck
- Footling

CLINICAL CONDITIONS PREDISPOSING TO BREECH

- Oligo/poly—extremes of amniotic fluid index (AFI)
- Multiple pregnancy
- Hydrocephaly/anencephaly
- Uterine anomalies
- Placenta previa
- Pelvic tumors
- Prior breech

Recurrence rate:

- 10% chances after 1 breech
- 28% after 2 breech delivery

Route of delivery depends on:

- Fetal breech type
- Maternal pelvis
- Existing morbidities
- Patient preference
- Hospital capability
- Provider skill and experience

Preterm breech has distinct complications than term breech.

- Head entrapment
- Birth trauma
- High-perinatal morbidity

Delivery complications:

- Injury to genital tract—cervix, vaginal wall
- Episiotomy incision extended
- Instrumental delivery
- Postpartum hemorrhage (PPH)
- Birth trauma—humerus, clavicle, and femur
- Brachial plexus injury
- Sternocleidomastoid hematoma

DIAGNOSIS

Made by abdominal examination: Head is felt on fundal grip, breech/podalic pole lies in LUS and fetal heart sound (FHS) heard at or little above umbilicus.

IMAGING

Fetal size and type of breech.

Factors favoring lower segment cesarean section (LSCS):

- Lack of expertise
- Patient request
- >3.8 kg/<1.2 kg or estimated fetal birth weight (EFBW) <10th percentile
- Apparently healthy/viable preterm fetus
- Severe fetal growth restriction (FGR) (EFBW <3rd percentile)
- Anomaly incompatible with vaginal delivery
- Prior prenatal/neonatal deaths
- Incomplete/footling breech
- Hyperextended neck on ultrasonography (USG)
- Previous LSCS
- Pelvis contracted or unfavorable

Vaginal delivery can be allowed if:

- Fetopelvic disproportion is ruled out
- No maternal complications, e.g., heart disease, severe preeclampsia, abruption, etc.
- Estimated fetal weight is 2–3.5 kg
- Favorable fetal attitude
- Availability of experienced obstetrician and pediatrician

RECOMMENDATIONS

In antenatal period, breech presentation at term should be offered external cephalic version (ECV) unless there is an absolute contraindication, between 35 and 37 weeks. If ECV unsuccessful or declined, counseling on risks and benefits of planned vaginal breech delivery versus planned LSCS. Planned LSCS leads to a small reduction in perinatal mortality compared with planned vaginal breech delivery, due to three reasons—(1) avoidance of stillbirth >39 weeks of gestation, (2) avoidance of intrapartum risks, and (3) risks of vaginal breech birth.

Risk of perinatal mortality is 1/1,000 with cephalic delivery, 2/1,000 with vaginal breech delivery, and 5/10,000 with LSCS >39 weeks. ~40% of women planning a vaginal breech birth may need emergency LSCS during labor.

Intranatal Period

If an unplanned vaginal breech presents in labor, management depends on stage of labor, any complications present, availability of clinical expertise, and informed consent. If near or in active second stage of labor no routine LSCS. If time and circumstances permit, USG done for position of fetal neck and legs, and EFBW should be estimated.

Induction of labor not recommended. Augmentation of slow progress with Oxytocin can be done if contraction frequency is low (<4/10 minutes) in presence of epidural analgesia. Birth in hospital with facilities for immediate cesarean section is recommended with planned vaginal breech birth and continuous electronic fetal monitoring (CEFM), but birth in an OT not recommended. Adequate progress of labor in first stage and descent of the breech in passive second stage is a prerequisite for encouragement of active second stage. Assistance, without traction, if delay or evidence of poor fetal condition.

If breech is not visible within 2 hours of passive second stage, LSCS is recommended. Maternal effort should not start until breech is visible, with "hands off" approach. If there is no progress/back rotates away from anterior/ poor tone, extended arms, or an extended neck; or delay of >5 minutes from delivery of buttocks-to-head, or >3 minutes from umbilicus-to-head, intervention should be done. Tactile stimulation of fetus may result in reflex extension of arms or head, so should be minimized. Fetus grasped around the pelvic girdle (not soft tissues) and neck should never be hyperextended, with selective episiotomy. If back starts to rotate posteriorly, gentle rotation without traction done to ensure that it remains anterior.

Once scapula is visible, arms can be hooked down by inserting a finger in elbow and flexing the arms across chest or, if nuchal, Lovset's maneuver. Delivery of head by Mauriceau–Smellie–Veit maneuver or with forceps. Suprapubic pressure aid flexion of extended neck. Delivery using Burns–Marshall technique is **not** advised due to concern of over extension of the fetal neck.

Preterm Breech

Routine cesarean section for breech in spontaneous preterm labor not recommended (except maternal and/ or fetal compromise). The mode of delivery should be individualized based on the stage of labor, type of breech, fetal wellbeing, and availability of an operator skilled in vaginal breech delivery. Labor with a preterm breech should be managed as with a term breech. If head entrapment, incisions in the cervix (vaginal birth) or vertical uterine incision extension (cesarean section) may be used.

SUGGESTED READING

1. ACOG Committee Opinion CO Number 745: Mode of Term Singleton Breech Delivery. Obstet Gynecol. 2018; 132(2):e60-e63.
2. RCOG. (2017). Management of Breech Presentation (Green-top Guideline No. 20b). [online] Available from https://www.rcog.org.uk/guidance/browse-all-guidance/green-top-guidelines/management-of-breech-presentation-green-top-guideline-no-20b/ [Last accessed September, 2024].

CHAPTER 20

Cord Prolapse

DEFINITION

Descent of umbilical cord through the cervix alongside ***(occult**—slips to the side but not ahead)* or past (***overt**—slips ahead*) the fetal presenting part in presence of ruptured membranes.

CORD PRESENTATION

Presence *(floating)* of umbilical cord between the cervix and the fetal presenting part, with or without intact membranes.

Recently an alternative definition according to the positional relationship among cord, fetal presenting part, and cervix has been proposed—"cord prolapse" refers to cord being slipped past the presenting part and beyond internal cervical os; "cord presentation" refers to cord ahead of presenting part but still above internal cervical os; "compound cord presentation" refers to both cord and fetus presenting above internal cervical os; all with intact/ruptured membranes.

INCIDENCE

About 0.1–0.6% (1% in breech). An unpredictable obstetric emergency as it is responsible for high perinatal mortality (~25% in low-income countries to 10% in high-income countries) due to birth asphyxia, caused by cord compression and umbilical arterial and venous vasospasm.

RISK FACTORS

- *General:* Multigravidas, polyhydramnios, malpresentation (breech, transverse, oblique, or unstable lie), second twin, low birth weight (LBW), preterm labor, congenital fetal anomaly, high floating nonengaged fetal head in labor, low-lying placenta, long cord, and atypical placental-cord insertions—velamentous/marginal
- *Procedure related:* ARM with high floating head, external cephalic version (ECV), internal podalic version (IPV), vaginal manipulation, stabilizing induction, catheter large balloon induction of labor (IOL), amnio-infusion, application of scalp electrode/intrauterine pressure catheter, manual rotation of fetal head, and amnioreduction.

PREVENTION

In polyhydramnios/unstable lie/malpresentation—elective hospital admission >37 weeks/when labor pain starts/prelabor rupture of membranes (PROM) (term/preterm) occurs. Avoid ARM with high floating (nonengaged) head or when cord is felt below the presenting part; avoid upward pressure on the presenting part during pv examination or any obstetric intervention; LSCS for cord presentation in established labor.

DIAGNOSIS

- *Antepartum:* Real-time USG + color Doppler may show the cord interposed between fetal presenting part and internal cervical os, especially in malpresentation.
- *Intrapartum:* Suspected if abrupt onset of severe prolonged bradycardia/moderate-to-severe variable decelerations/prolonged deceleration >1 minute, after a previously normal tracing, in presence of risk factors. Per speculum and per vaginal examination done to rule out overt cord prolapse, diagnosed on visualization/palpation of cord ahead of presenting part.
- *Differential diagnosis of fetal heart changes:* Fall of maternal BP (spinal anesthesia), tachysystole (uterine contraction >5 in 10 minutes), abruptio, and rupture uterus/vasa previa.

MANAGEMENT

Intrapartum

If the cord has no pulsation, fetal heart rate (FHR) should be confirmed immediately by stethoscope/Doppler, and USG, if dead then management depends on presentation, uterine contraction, and cervical status.

If found alive then definite treatment is prompt delivery to prevent fetal death from cord compression, if alive. Call for help → declare obstetric emergency → alert anesthesia, OT, pediatrician and nurses → initiate maneuvers for intrauterine resuscitation, minimize cord handling and avoid exposing to cold (vasospasm) → continuous monitoring of FHR → perform emergency delivery by most rapid and safe method, i.e., instrumental (forceps/ventouse) vaginal delivery if in second stage of full cervical dilatation fetus can be delivered safely and/or more quickly than lower segment cesarean section (LSCS), taking care to avoid impingement of the cord when possible.

But if in first stage of labor/before full dilatation of cervix—LSCS should be offered (depending on FHR tracing LSCS, may be category—I <30 minutes if FHR is pathological/category—II if FHR is normal with continuous monitoring and convert to category I if abnormal), along with intrauterine resuscitation → minimal handling of cord to prevent from vasospasm, manually elevate the presenting part, keep the patient in Trendelenburg/knee-chest position/exaggerated Sims position, i.e., left lateral (preferably with head down and pillow under the left hip), retrofilling the bladder by 500 mL NS and tocolytics [Terbutaline 250 μg SC (subcutaneous)] if abnormal FHR with contraction till LSCS done.

After delivery, delayed cord clamping only if baby is uncompromised but if compromised immediate cord clamping. A pediatrician competent in the neonatal resuscitation should be present in all deliveries of cord prolapse and paired cord blood samples should be sent for pH and base excess.

Documentation and explanation to patients and relatives.

OUTCOME

Single most important predictive factor of poor fetal outcome is the place where cord prolapse occurs—perinatal mortality is significantly more when it occurs outside the hospital (38–44%) as compared to within hospital (0–3%).

SUGGESTED READING

1. RCOG. (2014). Umbilical Cord Prolapse (Green-top Guideline No. 50). [online] Available from https://www.rcog.org.uk/guidance/browse-all-guidance/green-top-guidelines/umbilical-cord-prolapse-green-top-guideline-no-50/#:~:text=Cord%20prolapse%20has%20been%20defined,with%20or%20without%20membrane%20rupture. [Last accessed September, 2024].
2. Wong L, Kwan AHW, Lau SL, Sin WTA, Leung TY. Umbilical cord prolapse: revisiting its definition and management. Am J Obstet Gynecol. 2021;225(4):357-66.

CHAPTER 21

Shoulder Dystocia

DEFINITION

It is a complication of vaginal delivery in which shoulder of the fetus fails to deliver after the head has delivered with gentle downward axial traction, requiring additional obstetric maneuvers, i.e., head-to-body delivery time >60 seconds. Most commonly when anterior shoulder impacts on maternal symphysis, or less commonly when posterior shoulder impacts on sacral promontory.

INCIDENCE

About 0.2–3%, an obstetric emergency which can neither be predicted nor prevented.

RISK FACTORS

- Antepartum—diabetes mellitus (DM), obesity [body mass index (BMI) >30 kg/m^2], previous history of shoulder dystocia, estimated fetal birth weight (EFBW) >4.5 kg, and induction of labor (IOL)
- Intrapartum—prolonged first and second stage of labor, Oxytocin augmentation of labor, instrumental vaginal delivery, and precipitate labor.

Induction of labor at term in gestational diabetes mellitus (GDM) women with suspected macrosomia can reduce the incidence but not in nondiabetic women; elective lower segment cesarean section (LSCS) should be offered to diabetic women with EFBW ≥4.5 kg, and for nondiabetic women ≥5 kg.

DIAGNOSIS

Prompt recognition required if difficulty in delivering face and chin, failure of restitution, and head remains tightly opposed to vulva after delivery and sometimes it may retract inside ("turtle-neck" sign) and, shoulders fail to descend even after routine gentle axial traction in line of fetal spine, without any lateral traction.

MANAGEMENT

An obstetric emergency → call for help (senior gynecologist, experienced midwife, neonatal resuscitation team, anesthetist, nurses, and scriber) → explain to the patient, lie her flat and remove any back pillow (if used), and bring her to the edge of the table → "NO" to fundal pressure/maternal pushing → do McRobert's maneuver + suprapubic pressure (**first-line maneuver**). In McRobert's patient's thigh is hyperflexed on the abdomen with flexion and abduction of hips which straightens the lumbosacral angle and rotates maternal pelvis upward causing ↑ anteroposterior diameter of pelvis (90% success rate). Suprapubic pressure is applied by assistant with palm/fist from side of fetal back in downward and lateral direction just above the maternal symphysis pubis, which reduces the fetal bisacromial diameter and rotates the anterior shoulder into the wider oblique pelvic diameter. Gentle traction applied along with first maneuver to deliver the shoulder for 30 seconds each, if not then move to second maneuver.

Second-line maneuver—internal maneuver with episiotomy whole hand entered posteriorly to deliver posterior arm by grasping fetal wrist and gently withdrawing in straight line/perform internal rotation into an oblique diameter of maternal pelvis (or if possible, by a full 180° rotation of the fetal trunk) by applying pressure on the posterior aspect of the posterior shoulder which reduces the shoulder diameter by adducting the shoulder. If not successful then apply pressure on posterior aspect of the anterior shoulder to adduct and rotate the shoulders into maternal pelvic oblique diameter. Gentle axial traction applied along with to deliver for 30 seconds each, if no success then move the patient to "all fours" position and try to deliver the fetus for 30 seconds. If not successful then move to third-line maneuver.

Third-line maneuver—cleidotomy, i.e., surgical division of clavicle or bend with a finger, symphysiotomy, i.e., anterior fibers of pubic-symphysis ligament divided and the Zavanelli maneuver in which head is replaced vaginally and LSCS performed. Other techniques like use of a posterior axillary sling can be tried. There is low chance of hypoxic ischemic injury up to 5 minutes.

COMPLICATIONS

"NO" to fundal pressure as it may exacerbate impaction of the fetal shoulders and/or lead to uterine rupture. Second-line maneuvers, i.e., delivery of the posterior arm or internal rotation maneuvers are associated with fetal humeral fractures and brachial plexus injury (BPI). Third-line maneuvers are associated with serious maternal morbidity and poor neonatal outcome due to hypoxic-ischemic encephalopathy (HIE). Postpartum hemorrhage (PPH), obstetric anal sphincter injury (OASIS)—third and fourth degree perineal tears, cervicovaginal lacerations, trauma to urethra and bladder, uterine rupture, symphysis pubis diastasis, sacroiliac joint dislocation, and lateral femoral cutaneous neuropathy.

Neonatal injuries such as BPI, fracture humerus and clavicle, pneumothoraxes and HIE, besides soft tissue injuries, low APGAR, NICU admission, and ↑ perinatal morbidity and mortality.

Hence, proper training with simulation exercises and shoulder dystocia protocols is required to decrease complications and proper documentation to record significant facts, findings, and observations in order to decrease litigation.

Recurrence Rate

10%

SUGGESTED READING

1. Practice Bulletin Number 178: Shoulder Dystocia. Obstet Gynecol. 2017;129(5):e123-33.
2. RCOG. (2012). Shoulder Dystocia (Green-top Guideline No. 42). [online] Available from https://www.rcog.org.uk/guidance/browse-all-guidance/green-top-guidelines/shoulder-dystocia-green-top-guideline-no-42/ [Last accessed September, 2024].

CHAPTER 22

Antenatal Corticosteroids

BENEFITS

Benefits of antenatal corticosteroids if given within 7 days of preterm birth:

- Decrease perinatal death
- Decrease neonatal death
- Decrease respiratory distress syndrome
- Decrease intraventricular hemorrhage (IVH) and periventricular leukomalacia (23–24 weeks)
- Reduce developmental delay in childhood

Antenatal corticosteroids are most effective in reducing respiratory distress syndrome (RDS) in pregnancies if birth occurs between 24 hours and 7 days of administration of the second dose of antenatal corticosteroids.

It reduces neonatal (NN) deaths even if first dose given within 48 hours of birth, benefit is also seen even if birth is anticipated in next 24 hours. **No benefit** is seen if birth is >7 days after starting treatment. It affects maternal glucose tolerance (↑blood sugar) for 5 days after administration (with ↑risk in diabetics). No evidence that antenatal corticosteroids ↑ rates of maternal infection if given even in sepsis.

NICE Guideline recommends that planned lower segment cesarean section (LSCS) should not be carried out <39 weeks of gestation, but corticosteroids' role in planned cesarean birth at term (37–39 weeks) are:

- Reduce **admission to neonatal intensive care unit** (NICU) due to **respiratory morbidity**
- May cause harm to neonate—neonatal hypoglycemia and developmental delay (reduce educational attainment at school academics) if given in late pregnancy.
- Uncertain role in reduction of transient tachypnea of newborn (TTN), RDS, and **overall** NICU admission

Overall corticosteroids should be given from 24 weeks of gestation to 34^{+6} weeks gestation in:

- Established preterm labor
- Preterm premature rupture of membrane (PTPROM)
- Planned preterm birth
- Twins and triplets going for early birth

From 35^{+0} to 36^{+6} weeks, clinicians should weigh the risk benefit ratio as steroids have respiratory benefits, but increased risk of neonatal hypoglycemia is present.

Rescue course: If treatment given >7 days ago—reduces need for respiratory support, but also likely to ↓ birth weight, head circumference and length and NN blood pressure (BP).

ROLE OF CORTICOSTEROIDS IN MULTIPLE PREGNANCY

Effects are found to be no different than in singleton pregnancy, but single/multiple, untargeted (routine) administration of steroids should not be done.

Diabetes is **not** an absolute contraindication for antenatal corticosteroids. Additional insulin according to blood sugars should be given while administering corticosteroids in diabetic patients, as maternal blood sugar ↑ shortly after administration (elevated for 5 days) and ↑ NN hypoglycemia.

DOSAGE

- *Dexamethasone Phosphate* 6 mg 12 hourly—four doses intramuscular (↓IVH>)
- *Betamethasone Sodium Phosphate or Acetate* 12 mg 24 hourly—two doses intramuscular

RESCUE/REPEAT COURSE

A single repeat course of antenatal corticosteroids can be considered in women who are <34 weeks of gestation and are at risk of preterm delivery within next 7 days (especially if last dose given >7 days), as it reduces the need for neonatal respiratory support.

The maximum number of corticosteroid *courses* given in any one pregnancy should not exceed three (≥4 courses may be associated with the development of cerebral palsy). Babies who receive repeat doses of antenatal corticosteroids are smaller (lower birth weight and reduced length).

In the presence of systemic infection, the potential beneficial effects of antenatal corticosteroids intended for the baby are weighed against the effect of exacerbating the severity of systemic infection both for the woman and her baby.

SUGGESTED READING

1. Committee Opinion CO Number 713: Antenatal Corticosteroid Therapy for Fetal Maturation. Obstet Gynecol. 2017;130(2):e102-9.
2. RCOG. (2022). Antenatal corticosteroids to reduce neonatal morbidity and mortality (RCOG Green-top Guideline No. 74). [online] Available from https://www.rcog.org.uk/guidance/browse-all-guidance/green-top-guidelines/antenatal-corticosteroids-to-reduce-neonatal-morbidity-and-mortality-green-top-guideline-no-74/ [Last accessed September, 2024].

NOTES

SECTION 4

Medical and Surgical Disorders in Pregnancy

Section Authors: *Mridu Sinha, Jyoti Baghel, Babita Kumari, Saumya Agarwal*

CHAPTER 23

Anemia in Pregnancy

DEFINITION

Decrease in oxygen carrying capacity of blood to different tissues due to qualitative and/or quantitative deficiency of red blood cell (RBC)/hemoglobin (Hb)/both.

World Health Organization (WHO)—Hb concentration in peripheral blood <11 g/dL.

Center of Disease Control and Prevention (CDC): First trimester <11 g/dL ~ hematocrit (Hct) <33%; second trimester <10.5 g/dL ~ Hct <32%; third trimester <11 g/dL ~ Hct <33%; postpartum <10 g/dL ~ Hct <30%.

Indian Council of Medical Research Criteria (ICMR): Mild—Hb 10-10.9 g/dL, moderate—7-9.9 g/dL, severe—4-6.9 g/dL, and very severe <4 g/dL.

Modifiers of Hb concentration: High altitude, smoking, and medical condition such as preeclampsia.

PREVALENCE

In India, it is as high as 40-80% (WHO—high prevalence >40%, not problematic <5%). >50% of anemia is due to iron deficiency and approximately 20% of maternal death is due to anemia. Causes of high prevalence:

- Dietary habits—consumption of low bioavailability diets, phytates, tannates, and calcium
- Defective absorption—worm infestation, coeliac disease, and tropical sprue
- Low iron stores—low baseline reserves, multiple pregnancies and short interconceptional periods, menorrhagia, excessive sweating, and malaria.

PHYSIOLOGICAL (DILUTIONAL) ANEMIA DURING PREGNANCY

Mild, normocytic-normochromic diagnosis of exclusion (due to relative hemodilution Hb ↓ by approximately 2 g/dL). Blood volume in pregnancy starts to increase from 6th week (10-15%) and reaches maximum at 32 weeks. Plasma volume increases maximum up to 50% whereas RBC volume increases up to 20-30%.

IRON REQUIREMENT DURING PREGNANCY

Early pregnancy—2-3 mg/day, second trimester—4-6 mg/day, third trimester—6-8 mg/day, and average—4 mg/day. Iron absorption is increased from 7% in first trimester to 66% in third trimester. Factors enhancing absorption includes gastric acidity, ascorbic acid, vinegar, fermented food items and alcohol, low iron stores, and increased erythropoietin activity. Factors which inhibit absorption are phytates, oxalates, calcium, milk, and tea-coffee.

Stages of Development of Iron Deficiency Anemia

- Stage I—*storage* iron depletion (serum ferritin <30 ng/mL) (1 nanograms/milliliter = 1 micrograms/liter)
- Stage II—iron deficient erythropoiesis [ferrokinetic studies -↓Serum Fe, ↑ total iron binding capacity (TIBC), ↓transferrin saturation, ↑ zinc protoporphyrin (ZPP) and ↑soluble transferrin receptor assay] (storage + transport Fe)
- Stage III—iron deficiency anemia (GBP and Hb) (storage + transport + functional Fe)

APPROACH TO A CASE OF ANEMIA

- Clinical and laboratory assessment of severity of anemia
- Typing of anemia
- Finding cause of anemia
- Determining predisposing
- Precipitating factors

HISTORY TAKING

Worm infestation, bleeding per rectum (PR), hematuria, bleeding diathesis, pica, malnutrition, chronic disease such as TB, malaria, sickle cell anemia, pyelonephritis, malabsorption, excessive menstrual blood loss, and multiparity. Dietary history, any medication causing bone marrow suppression, family history, and residence of endemic areas.

- *C/F:*
  - Mild anemia—no adverse effect
  - Moderate anemia—fatigue, weakness, lassitude, exhaustion, anorexia, indigestion, dyspnea, giddiness, headache, and light-headedness
  - Severe anemia—tachycardia, dyspnea, palpitations, increased cardiac output, congestive heart failure, pulmonary edema, generalized anasarca, skin, and nail changes.
- *O/E:* Pallor, koilonychia (nail changes), cheilosis (swelling and fissuring of lips), glossitis (swollen and inflamed tongue), stomatitis (sore and inflamed mouth), alopecia, hyperdynamic circulation (short and soft systolic murmur), signs of congestive heart failure, i.e., tachycardia, tachypnoea, ↑ jugular venous pressure (JVP), ankle edema, and postural hypotension. Plummer-Vinson or Paterson-Kelly syndrome (dysphagia + esophageal webs), pica (eats chalk/soil), and pagophagia (eats ice).

MATERNAL COMPLICATIONS

- *During pregnancy:* Preeclampsia (30%), preterm labor, intercurrent infection, heart failure (30–32 weeks), and abruptio placenta
- *During labor:* Uterine inertia, postpartum hemorrhage (PPH), cardiac failure, and shock
- *During puerperium:* Puerperal sepsis, subinvolution, lactation failure, venous thromboembolism (VTE), and delayed wound healing.

Fetal Risks

Prematurity, low birth weight (LBW), fetal death, increased perinatal morbidity and mortality, anemia in infancy, behavioral abnormality, poor performance, and poor cognitive functions.

INVESTIGATIONS

- Peripheral smear—microcytic, hypochromic RBC, mean corpuscular volume (MCV), mean corpuscular hemoglobin (MCH), and mean corpuscular hemoglobin concentration (MCHC) ↓
- ↓Serum iron is low <60 µg/dL (60–120), ↓serum ferritin <30 µg/L or ng/mL (30–150) (serum ferritin is a sensitive marker for iron deficiency, but not very specific as it is an acute phase reactant and may be increased in infection, inflammation, and malignancy, thereby masking Fe deficiency. 1 ng/mL of serum ferritin equivalent to 8 mg of storage iron).

TABLE 1: Main differences between iron deficiency anemia and thalassemia.

d/d between	*Fe deficiency anemia*	*Thalassemia*
MCHC	↓	N
RDW	>15%	N
HbF	N (<2%)	>2%
HbA2	N (2–3%)	>3.5%
FEP	↑	N
Mentzer index (MCV/RBC)	>13	<13

(FEP: erythrocyte porphyrin; HbA2: hemoglobin A2; HbF: fetal hemoglobin; MCV: mean corpuscular volume; MCHC: mean corpuscular hemoglobin concentration; RBC: red blood cell; RDW: red cell distribution width)

- ↑TIBC is increased >400 µg/dL (325–400)
- ↓Transferrin saturation (Serum Fe/TIBC) <15% (20–50)
- ↑Erythrocyte ZPP >40–70 µmol/mol heme
- ↑Serum transferrin receptor(↑threefold to fivefold), ↑serum transferrin receptor: Serum ferritin index (anemia-chronic disease <1) (Fe deficiency anemia >2)
- Reticulocyte indices:
  - Mentzer index—MCV/RBC count (Fe deficiency anemia >13) (thalassemia <13)
  - ↑(RDW >15%) red cell distribution width to d/d between Fe deficiency anemia and thalassemia

Table 1 shows the main differences between iron deficiency anemia and thalassemia.

PREVENTION

Dietary modifications—↑green leafy veg, sprouts, peas, jaggery, dried fruits (apricot), liver, meat, and eggs. Iron supplementation of adolescent (12 × 12 Govt. of India initiative and nonpregnant women of childbearing age), in pregnant women, treatment of hookworm infection, food fortification. ANC for early recognition and prompt treatment of Fe deficiency.

MANAGEMENT

- General treatment—diet rich in iron, proteins, vitamins and ascorbic acid, elimination of septic foci, checking compliance to therapy. **Flowchart 1** shows how to approach a case of anemia in pregnancy.
- Specific treatment—choice of therapy depends on gestational age and severity of anemia. WHO recommends 60 mg elemental Fe + 400 µg Folic acid/day for 6 months where prevalence <40% and this dose

Flowchart 1: Approach to a case of anemia in pregnancy.

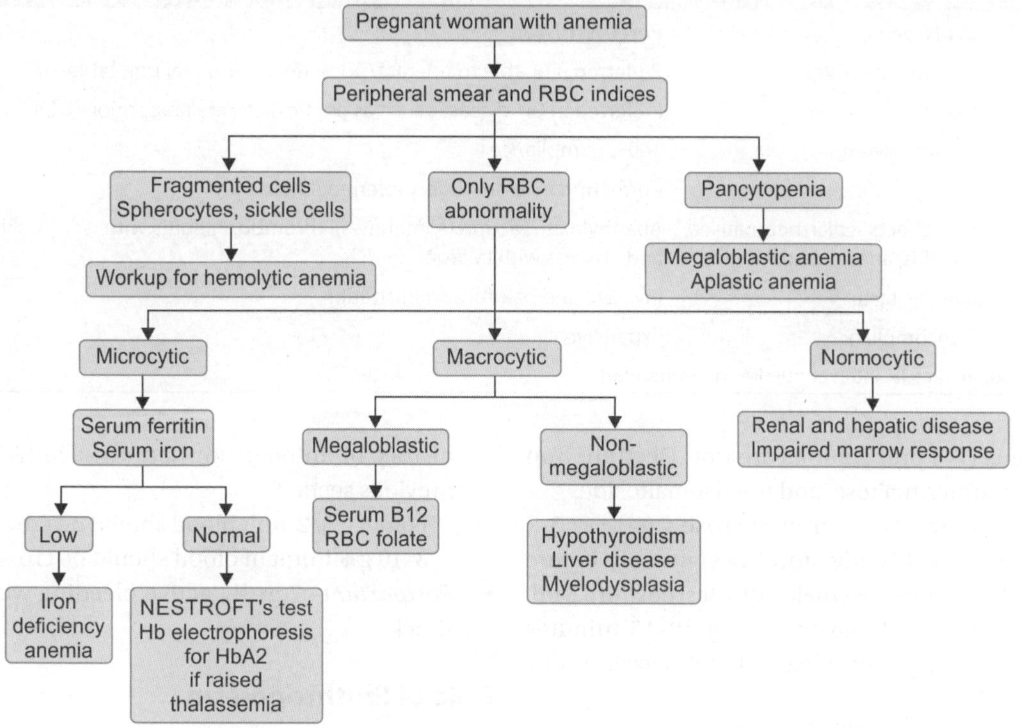

(HbA2: hemoglobin A2; NESTROFT: naked eye single tube red cell osmotic fragility test; RBC: red blood cell)

supplemented for another 3 months postpartum where prevalence >40%. To maximize absorption, iron tablets should be taken at night or at least 1 hour prior/after food. National Nutritional Anemia Control Program of India recommends 100 mg elemental Fe + 500 µg Folic acid for at least 100 days, starting in second trimester for prophylaxis and double this dose for treatment, and should be continued for next 3 months to build up the stores. Side-effects—nausea, vomiting, abdominal discomfort, constipation, and dark stools due to free iron radical-mediated gastrointestinal tract (GIT) mucosal damage.

Response to Treatment

- Clinical improvement—symptoms improvement, increase sense of well-being and increase work capacity.
- Laboratory parameters within 5–7 days ↑ reticulocyte count to 5% (N = 0.2–2%)
  - 2–3 weeks—↑ Hb level 0.8–1 g/dL/week, improved—MCV, MCH, and MCHC
  - 6–8 weeks—Hb level comes to normal level, ↑serum ferritin level and GBP show normocytic normochromic RBCs.

Reasons for Failure to Respond

Noncompliant patient, coexisting folate deficiency, infection, continuous blood loss, hookworm infestation, bleeding hemorrhoids, faulty iron absorption, and inaccurate diagnosis—noniron deficiency microcytic anemia.

Indications of Parenteral Iron

Intolerance to oral iron or causing side-effects, impaired iron absorption, chronic blood loss, and gastrointestinal disorders such as peptic ulcer, ulcerative colitis [inflammatory bowel disease (IBD)], >32 weeks of gestation, preferred as compliance is 100%. Maximum rise in hemoglobin achievable with either oral or parenteral iron is 0.8 g/dL/week. Intramuscular injection are not used due to unpredictability of allergic reaction, local irritation at injection site, skin discoloration, and possibly sarcomatous change. IV injections are given in hospital due to chance of anaphylaxis (sudden onset respiratory difficulty and/or cardiovascular collapse) and oral iron should be discontinued before it as receptors are choked leading to increased risk of toxicity from free circulatory

TABLE 2: Main differences between oral iron and parenteral iron.

	Oral iron	*Parenteral iron*
Advantages	Easy to administer	Preferred if unable to tolerate/side-effects with oral iron tablets
	Cheap	Preferred in GIT diseases such as peptic ulcer, malabsorption (UC/CD/tropical sprue)
	No anaphylaxis	100% compliance
		Correction in lesser time, preferred if near term
Disadvantages	Side effects—diarrhea, nausea, gastritis, and constipation	Anaphylaxis reaction (sometimes), thrombophlebitis with IV iron, skin staining, and abscess with IM iron
	Metallic taste	Invasive and painful administration
	Noncompliance	Expensive

(GIT: gastrointestinal tract; IV: intravenous; IM: intramuscular)

Fe. intravenous (IV) preparations are iron Dextran, iron Sucrose, iron Carboxymaltose, and Iron Isomaltoside.

Dose calculation (TDI)—iron Sucrose (mg) = 2.3 × weight × deficit + 500 (body store) [weight (kg) before pregnancy, deficit = target—actual(g/dL)] test dose of 0.5 mL (25 mg diluted in 50 mL) given IV over 10–15 minutes and full dose after a lapse of at least 1 hour to exclude any reaction.

Ferric Carboxymaltose (FCM) has certain advantages—no test dose required, can be given by bolus IV injection or fast IV infusion and usually not associated with anaphylactic reaction.

Table 2 displays the relative advantages-disadvantages of oral Vs parenteral iron therapy.

BLOOD TRANSFUSION

Each unit of packed RBCs transfused raises Hb by 1 g/dL. Side effects—fluid overload [transfusion-associated circulatory overload (TACO)], anaphylaxis, allergic reaction, acute lung injury [transfusion-related acute lung injury (TRALI)], infection, and potential sensitization of RBC antigen. According to FOGSI guidelines, the indications of blood transfusion are:

- *Antepartum:*
  - <34 weeks—Hb ≤5 g/dL or Hb 5–7 g/dL with signs of cardiac failure, hypoxia, pneumonia, malaria, or any other bacterial infection
  - 34 weeks or more—Hb ≤7 g/dL or 6–8 g/dL with signs of cardiac failure, hypoxia, pneumonia, malaria, or any other bacterial infection
  - Acute hemorrhage leading to shock/<6 g/dL, hemoglobinopathy, and bone marrow failure
- *Intrapartum: <7 g/dL in labor, any medical condition leading to severe anemia, bleeding*: Elective LSCS with history of antepartum hemorrhage (APH), PPH, or previous section.

  For <8 g%, 2-unit blood should be cross matched 8–10 g% 1 unit of blood should be cross matched.
- *Postpartum* <7 g/dL, active bleeding with features of shock

Role of Erythropoietin

- Erythropoietin—glycoprotein with 165 amino acids, molecular weight 55,000 kD, half-life 2–4 hours, secreted by renal peritubular interstitial cells in response to decreased oxygen tension.
- Acts by binding to erythropoietin receptors on erythroblasts in bone marrow and increase Hb synthesis in 12 hours and increase RBC counts by four to five times within 2 weeks.
- Indicated in iron deficiency anemia, anemia of chronic disease, and in end-stage renal disease with anemia, dose—100–150 IU/kg three times a week subcutaneously.
- Side effects—hypertension, thrombosis, myalgia, seizures, and flu-like symptoms.

SUGGESTED READING

1. Arias F, Bhide AG, Arulkumaran S, Damania K, Daftary SN, editors. Arias' practical guide to high-risk pregnancy and delivery: A south Asian perspective. 5th edition. New Delhi, India: Elsevier; 2019.
2. FOGSI. Guidelines for clinical practice recommendations on management of iron deficiency anemia in pregnancy. 2016. Available from: https://www.fogsi.org/wp-content/uploads/2016/05/The-evidence-base_IDA-Pregnancy-24-May-2016-Clean.pdf.
3. Misra R (Ed). Ian Donald's Practical Obstetrics Problems. 8th edition. India: Wolters Kluwer; 2020.

CHAPTER 24

Thrombocytopenia in Pregnancy

INTRODUCTION

Normally platelet counts decrease 15–20% during uncomplicated pregnancies, but usually remain in normal range, i.e., 1.5–4.5 lakhs/μL.

DEFINITION

Platelet count below the lower limit of normal range, i.e., <1.5 lakhs/μL. Mild thrombocytopenia—1 to <1.5 lakhs/μL, moderate—50 thousand–1 lakh/μL, Severe—<50,000/μL blood.

INCIDENCE

8–10%. *Causes:* 75% gestational (GT) thrombocytopenia, 15–20% hypertensive disorders, 3–4% immune process, and 1–2% constitutional, infections, and hematological malignancies.

- *Gestational (GT)/incidental thrombocytopenia*—self-limited condition, diagnosis of exclusion; 8–10% of all pregnancies and 75% of thrombocytopenia in pregnancy; usually mild type with platelet count >70,000; occurs in third trimester, not associated with maternal bleeding/bruising and/or fetal thrombocytopenia, no previous history of thrombocytopenia outside pregnancy [as compared to immune thrombocytopenia (ITP)], spontaneous resolution after delivery (6 weeks) but may recur in subsequent pregnancies. Exact cause not known but thought to be accelerated destruction/pooling/consumption of platelets across the placenta apart from physiological hemodilution. Management—on investigation (or clinical examination) no abnormality in blood tests, no treatment required, and no change in antenatal care/delivery. Periodic monitoring of platelet counts, and if <80,000 → anesthetic review, no fetal blood sampling (FBS)/fetal scalp electrodes, no midcavity, or high operative vaginal delivery, send cord blood sample and neonatal sample on D1 and D4 to rule out neonatal thrombocytopenia.
- *Immune thrombocytopenic purpura (ITP):* Chronic condition, also diagnosis of exclusion but in majority of cases diagnosed before pregnancy; cause—antibodies specific to platelet surface glycoproteins bind to platelets in the maternal circulation, resulting in immune-mediated platelet destruction; also, can cross placenta and cause fetal thrombocytopenia. Besides, there is also suppression of platelet production; 0.1–1/1,000 pregnancies. Mostly asymptomatic but few may have epistaxis/mucous membrane bleeding, and hematuria/gastrointestinal tract (GIT) bleeding. Management—combined obstetric/hematology clinic, Prednisolone first-line medication, started at lower dose of 20 mg (as compared to nonpregnant) to minimize the risk of adverse effects—gestational diabetes mellitus (GDM) and postpartum psychoses. If no response, IV immunoglobulin/anti-D, splenectomy, and platelet transfusion done.
- *Hypertensive disorders of pregnancy*—preeclampsia (PE) [5–10% pregnancy, characterized by ↑ blood pressure (BP) and proteinuria/end-organ dysfunction], PE with severe features [BP ≥160/110, new-onset cerebral/visual disturbances—headache, epigastric pain, photopsia, scotomata, and cortical blindness; abnormal liver function test (LFT)], eclampsia; hemolysis, elevated liver enzymes, and low platelet count (HELLP) syndrome; PE associated with microangiopathic hemolytic anemia [MAHA—schistocytes in peripheral blood smear (PBS), ↑ lactic dehydrogenase (LDH), ↑bilirubin, and ↓haptoglobin].
- *Disseminated intravascular coagulation (DIC)*—massive activation of coagulation and fibrinolysis within vascular system, leading to depletion of clotting factors [↑prothrombin time/activated partial thromboplastin time (PT/APTT), ↓Fibrinogen, and ↑D-dimer] and ↓platelets with ↑risk of severe bleeding. Causes—abruptio, retained intrauterine fetal demise (IUFD), sepsis, amniotic fluid embolism, etc.
- *Acute fatty liver of pregnancy (AFLP)*—uncommon liver injury in third trimester, fatty infiltration of liver

cause of deranged LFT (±↑PT/APTT and ↓fibrinogen), nausea, vomiting, and pain abdomen.

- *Thrombotic microangiopathy (TMA)*—conditions in which platelet microthrombi form in small vessels leading to organ damage, MAHA, and ↓platelets:
    - *Thrombotic thrombocytopenic purpura (TTP)*—associated with ↓ADAMTS13 activity ± neurologic manifestations. [ADAMTS13 is a protein that regulates coagulation by cleaving von Willebrand factor (vWF) multimers into smaller, inactive fragments]. Treatment—plasma exchange and/or infusion (hereditary).
    - *Complement-mediated TMA*—associated with activation of complement system of endothelial cells leading to microthrombi in small blood vessels especially of kidney [acute kidney injury (AKI)]. Treatment—anticomplement therapy.
    - *Shiga toxin-mediated hemolytic-uremic syndrome (HUS)*—enteric infection (*E. coli* and *Shigella*) produces toxin leading to TMA, severe abdominal pain associated with bloody diarrhea ± fever and neurologic symptoms, accompanied by renal insufficiency. Treatment—antibiotics.
- Other causes—systemic lupus erythematosus (SLE), antiphospholipid syndrome (APS), drug-induced immune thrombocytopenic purpura/Heparin-induced thrombocytopenia/TMA (ITP/HIT/TMA), infections [dengue, malaria, human immunodeficiency virus (HIV), hepatitis C virus (HCV), etc.], liver disease, deficiency of vitamin B_{12}/Cu/FA; inherited platelet disorders, type 2B von Willebrand disease (vWD), and cancers.

EVALUATION

History of any complications, infection (fever and chills), medications, obstetric history, personal or family history of bleeding diathesis, autoimmune disease/liver disease, severity of anemia, course of pregnancy, timing of platelet drop, and abnormalities of PBS.

MANAGEMENT

Multidisciplinary team (MDT) from maternal-fetal medicine, hematology, nephrology, and microbiologist. If platelet count between 1 and 1.5 lakh/μL (mild), without any C/F or cytopenia, likely to be GT/ITP (both diagnosis of exclusion) needs observation with frequent monitoring of platelet count, and if asymptomatic isolated thrombocytopenia <1 lakh/μL then ITP more likely. If history and/or examination suggest cause other than GT/ITP, then treatment of cause. If symptomatic thrombocytopenia <1 lakh/μL, with bleeding/thrombosis/any C/F then investigate for all causes including complete blood count (CBC), general blood picture (GBP), PT/APTT/international normalized ratio (INR), fibrinogen, red blood cell (RBC) indices, liver function tests/renal function tests (LFT/RFT), lactate dehydrogenase (LDH), etc.

Delivery—if the cause is pregnancy-induced, then plan delivery and during delivery avoid forceps/ventouse, FBS, or fetal scalp electrodes to prevent intracranial hemorrhage (ICH) in fetus (in case fetal thrombocytopenia). Cord blood should be sent to rule out neonatal thrombocytopenia and avoid IM vitamin K until platelet count is known.

Role of platelet transfusion—if <20,000/μL or associated with severe bleeding episodes, aim for 30,000/μL for vaginal delivery, 50,000/μL for LSCS/major surgeries, and >80,000/μL for spinal/epidural anesthesia.

RECURRENCE

↑with GT, ITP, and hereditary TTP.

SUGGESTED READING

1. Myers B. Thrombocytopenia in pregnancy. Obstet Gynaecol. 2009;11:177-83.
2. Practice Bulletin Number 207: Thrombocytopenia in Pregnancy. Obstet Gynecol. 2019;133(3):e181-93.

CHAPTER 25

Rheumatic Heart Disease in Pregnancy

Overall incidence is 1–3%.

TYPES

- Congenital
- Acquired

Ischemic heart disease (IHD) in developed countries, rheumatic heart disease (RHD) in developing countries, and cardiomyopathies. Mitral stenosis (MS) is the most common RHD in developing countries.

MITRAL STENOSIS

Thickening (due to fibrosis, fusion, and calcification) and immobility of mitral valves (chordae tendineae) causing obstruction in blood flow from left atrium to left ventricle, leading to ↑backpressure in left atrium, pulmonary vessels, and right heart. Most common cause is rheumatic fever (inflammation of valve leaflets due to cross-reactivity between Group Aβ-hemolytic streptococcal antigen and valve tissues). In absence of correction, it is usually a progressive condition from asymptomatic (stage A) to symptomatic (B and C) [four stages—A (asymptomatic, at risk), B (progressive), C (asymptomatic, severe), and D (symptomatic severe)]. Valve area <2.5 cm^2 causes dyspnea on exertion and <1.5 cm^2 produces symptom at rest. Incidence: 0.1–4%.

Effect of Pregnancy on Mitral Stenosis

Due to ↑heart rate and cardiac output, patient becomes symptomatic/exacerbation of symptoms in symptomatic. Complications include atrial fibrillation, atrial flutter, supraventricular tachycardia, secondary pulmonary hypertension (HTN), tricuspid regurgitation, heart failure (30–32 weeks, labor, PP), and systemic thromboembolism. Cause of death are right heart failure [↑jugular venous pressure (JVP), tender hepatomegaly, and ankle edema] and/or pulmonary edema.

Effect of Mitral Stenosis on Pregnancy

Effect of MS on pregnancy are preterm labor and prematurity, low birth weight (LBW) [fetal growth restriction (FGR) in cyanotic heart disease], and perinatal death.

Symptoms

Symptoms are progressive exertional dyspnea, orthopnea, hemoptysis, fatigue, palpitations, nocturnal cough, exercise intolerance, syncope, and chest pain.

Signs

Signs are ↑JVP, cyanosis, clubbing, on auscultation-pansystolic murmur/late systolic murmur, loud systolic murmur >grade 3, diastolic murmur with thrill, loud ejection systolic murmur, splitting of second heart sound, and basal crepitations.

Diagnostic Tools

Chest X-ray posteroanterior (PA) view with shield (cardiomegaly, ↑pulmonary vascular markings), electrocardiography (ECG) (T-wave inversion, atrial enlargement, and arrhythmias), two-dimensional echocardiography (2D-ECHO) [left ventricular ejection fraction (LVEF), and valve area >1.5 cm^2 → mild, 1–1.5 cm^2 → moderate, and <1 cm^2 → severe] are diagnostic tools. New York Heart Association (NYHA) functional assessment.

MANAGEMENT

High-risk pregnancy (HRP), multidisciplinary team (MDT)—cardiologist, obstetrician (expertise maternal-fetal medicine), anesthetist, pediatrician, specialist nurse, and whole cardiac team. CVS risk assessment and prevent cardiac failure, cessation of teratogenic medications [Angiotensin receptor blocker/Angiotensin-converting enzyme (ARBs/ACE)-inhibitors/Warfarin].

Antenatal Care

Antenatal visit every 2 weeks till 30 weeks, thereafter weekly till delivery. At each visit, enquire about symptoms—dyspnea/limitation of activity, rest is advised and avoid undue exertion, Iron + Folic acid + Calcium supplementation, early diagnosis, and treatment of risk factors for cardiac failure—infections (dental/respiratory infection), anemia, arrhythmias, HTN, and hyperthyroidism; all women with RHD should receive Penicillin prophylaxis (Benzathine penicillin) to avoid bacterial endocarditis. Beta-blocker/Digitalis if tachycardia, low dose Furosemide, and anticoagulation with Low-molecular-weight Heparin (LMWH) (discontinue in labor). Cardiac intervention if not responding to medical management/severe MS—percutaneous mitral balloon valvotomy. Antenatal fetal surveillance.

Peripartum

Discuss timing (spontaneous/induced), site of delivery (with cardiac facilities), route of delivery (vaginal/CS-reserved for obstetric/fetal indications/severe MS with valve area <1 cm^2, with heart failure/complications).

- *During first stage of labor:* Rest in semi-recumbent position, intravenous (IV) fluids should be avoided or restricted to 50–75 mL/h, intermittent O_2 at the rate of 5–6 L/min (grade three-fourths disease), analgesia, cardiac monitoring and pulse oximetry (±CVP), and prophylactic IV antibiotics—injection Ampicillin 2 g + injection Gentamicin 1.5 mg/kg at labor onset and repeated 8 hourly
- *During second stage of labor:* No maternal pushing and cut short second stage by assisted vaginal delivery by outlet forceps preferred over ventouse under pudendal/perineal block
- *During third stage of labor:* Injection Oxytocin 10 IU IM at delivery of placenta except in left to right shunt or severe outflow obstruction, single dose of IV Frusemide 20–40 mg, no Ergometrine to prevent sudden overloading of heart, No Prostaglandin F2α (PGF-2α), Misoprostol 1,000 μg PR to control postpartum hemorrhage (PPH).

Puerperium

Managed meticulously and close observation for 24 hours, 1–2 hours postdelivery "Golden Hour"—heart rate/respiratory rate/blood pressure (HR/RR/BP)—hourly recording, oxygen, breastfeeding allowed except when the patient is in heart failure. Follow-up at 4–6 weeks, then at 6 months.

Prognosis

Guarded if previous cardiac failure/arrhythmia/transient ischemic attack (TIA); NYHA III/IV; and LVEF <40%, moderate-to-severe degree of MS with features of left heart obstruction.

Contraception

Depot Medroxyprogesterone Acetate/Progestin-Only Pill (DMPA/POP)/Implanon can be given [CI—steroidal combined oral contraceptive (COC) due to thromboembolism and intrauterine contraceptive device (IUCD) due to infection], barrier best, and sterilization if family complete.

Preconception Care

MDT with cardiologist and gynecologist. Risk stratification by CARPREG-II score (based on 10 predictors)/modified World Health Organization (WHO) classification system/DEVI score. Counseling regarding complications, functional assessment, treatment of infection/anemia, safer medications (ACE inhibitors/ARBs should be changed) (Warfarin should be changed to Heparin as soon as pregnancy is confirmed~6 weeks) and suitable contraception till patient considered fit for pregnancy, any required cardiac intervention before conception—balloon valvotomy, mitral valve repair/replacement. MTP—Eisenmenger's syndrome, primary pulmonary HTN, cor pulmonale, single ventricle, and NYHA class III/IV likely to deteriorate in pregnancy.

PERIPARTUM CARDIOMYOPATHY

Definition (Diagnosis of Exclusion)

Idiopathic cardiomyopathy presenting with heart failure secondary to left ventricular systolic dysfunction (LVEF <45%) at the end of pregnancy or up to 6 months postpartum, with no other cause of heart failure (by ESC, 2010).

Risk Factors

Advanced maternal age, multiparity, multiple pregnancy, obesity, chronic HTN, preeclampsia, and ethnicity (Afro-Caribbean).

Etiology

Multifactorial, "two-hit" model of pathogenesis, wherein a vascular insult secondary to hormonal effects of advanced pregnancy causes cardiomyopathy in women with underlying genetic predisposition (genes that regulate myocyte function undergo mutation). When ↓STAT3 → ↑reactive oxidative species (ROS) →↑cathepsin D → cleaves prolactin into 16-kDa fragment→ ↑ cardiac endothelial and capillary dysfunction.

Clinical Features

Symptoms—dyspnea, orthopnea, paroxysmal nocturnal dyspnea (PND), unexplained cough (particularly when lying down ± frothy pink sputum), palpitations, dizziness, edema legs, abdominal discomfort caused by hepatic congestion, precordial pain, and fatigue. Signs—signs of heart failure—sinus tachycardia, ↑JVP, and basal lung crepitations; third heart sound, displaced apex beat.

Differential Diagnosis

Benign dyspnea of pregnancy, other heart disease—RHD (MS and AS), myocardial infarction (MI), arrhythmias, ischemic heart disease (atherosclerosis, coronary dissection, vasospasm, and coronary embolism), hypertensive heart disease, human immunodeficiency virus (HIV) cardiomyopathy, pulmonary embolism, and amniotic fluid embolism.

Approach

- *History:* Known congenital or acquired heart disease (?) Family history—ischemic/nonischemic heart disease (?)
- *Physical examination:* Tachypnea, tachycardia, peripheral edema, and ↑JVP
- *Electrocardiogram:* No specific pattern in peripartum cardiomyopathy (PPCM)—sinus tachycardia, nonspecific ST-segment, and T-wave abnormalities, but may rule out ischemic or thromboembolic cause.
- *Echocardiography:* It is crucial in diagnosing PPCM. LVEF <45%, ventricles may or may not be dilated [left ventricular end-diastolic diameter (LVEDD) >6 cm and LVEF <30% → poor prognosis and ↑mechanical support, transplant, and death]
- *Blood tests:* Hemoglobin ↓, ↑C reactive protein, ↑white cell count, ↑natriuretic peptides—Brain Natriuretic Peptide (BNP >100 pg/mL) or N-terminal pro-Brain Natriuretic Peptide (NT-pro BNP >300 pg/mL), Troponin T (WNL), and blood gas analysis if unstable.
- *Other investigations:* Chest X-ray (cardiac strain—alveolar shadowing, septal lines, cardiomegaly, pulmonary edema, and pleural effusion), cardiac magnetic resonance imaging (MRI) (assess cardiac chamber volume, systolic function, intracardiac thrombus, cardiac tissue injury—intracellular and interstitial injury, hyperemia, capillary leakage, necrosis, and fibrosis), and endomyocardial biopsy.

Management

High-risk pregnancy, MDT—obstetrician, cardiologist, neonatologist, anesthetist, and intensive care unit (ICU) intensivist. Assess heart failure severity: Systolic blood pressure (SBP) <90 mm Hg; HR >130/min or <45/min; RR >25/min; SpO_2 <90%; lactate >2.0 mmol/L; $ScvO_2$ <60%; altered mental state, cold skin; oliguria → severe acute heart failure/cardiogenic shock → ICU admission

- *Optimize oxygenation:* Prop-up position, oxygen by mask/noninvasive ventilation (NIV) + continuous positive airway pressure (CPAP), invasive ventilation with intubation if SpO_2 <95% despite all therapy
- *Maintain optimal preload:* Volume versus IV loop diuretics (Frusemide), IV vasodilators (Nitrates) if SBP >110 mm Hg
- *Add beta-blockers:* Selective β-antagonists, such as Metoprolol
- *Circulatory support:* Inotropes and/or vasopressors, Consider Levosimendan 0.1 μg/kg/min.
- *Consider Bromocriptine:* Dopamine D_2 agonist 2.5 mg once daily for at least 1 week (extended treatment—2.5 mg BD for 2 weeks, then 2.5 mg OD for 6 weeks when ejection fraction <25%, with or without associated cardiogenic shock)
- Anticoagulation with LMWH
- Consider mechanical circulatory support
- Antepartum →fetal growth monitoring with serial growth scans, in severe cases → urgent delivery (timing of delivery balanced between deteriorating maternal condition and fetal prematurity), induction of labor (IOL) for obstetric indication or for deteriorating cardiac function, lower segment cesarean section (LSCS) for an obstetric reason or if there is severe maternal compromise; IM corticosteroids between 24 weeks of gestation and 35^{+6} weeks gestational age to promote fetal lung maturation.

- Intrapartum—continuous electronic fetal monitoring (CEFM), hourly monitoring of fluid balance, BP, pulse, respiratory rate, oxygen saturation, continuous ECG, 30° left tilt to avoid aortocaval compression, low-dose regional analgesia, and cut short second stage with instrumental delivery, in third-stage low infusion Oxytocin as first line to prevent PPH (second line—Misoprostol and Carboprost) (no Ergometrine/Carbetocin)
- *Heart failure therapy:* Hydralazine, nitrates, beta-blocker, diuretics [postpartum—heart failure therapy: ACE-I (or ARB), beta-blocker, mineralocorticoid receptor (MR) antagonist, diuretics, consider Bromocriptine]
- Consider cardioversion/defibrillator if LVEF ≤35%
- *Breastfeeding:* Continue except when symptomatic and hemodynamically unstable, or if the LVEF <45%, breastfeeding avoided

Prognosis

50–80% recovers, mortality is 10%. Recurrence risk—20% if complete recovery but ↑50% with persistent left ventricular dysfunction (20% risk of mortality).

Contraception

Long-acting reversible contraception (LARC) [IUCD, Levonorgestrel intrauterine system (LNG-IUS), DMPA, and implant] (IUCD should be fitted in hospital with adequate resuscitation facility due to risk of vasovagal collapse) and POP safe (COC-CI), barrier (↑failure), and sterilization (anesthetic risks).

SUGGESTED READING

1. Kulkarni A, Squire G, Hogrefe K, Waseem Osman M. Peripartum cardiomyopathy. The Obstetrician and Gynaecologist. 2021;23:278-89.
2. Nelson-Piercy C. Handbook of Obstetric Medicine. 5th edition. Boca Raton: CRC Press; 2015. p. 36.

CHAPTER 26

Gestational Diabetes Mellitus

INTRODUCTION

Gestational diabetes mellitus (GDM) is defined as carbohydrate intolerance of variable severity, resulting in hyperglycemia with onset or first recognition during pregnancy. Prevalence in India—13%.

CLASSIFICATION

- *Type 1 diabetes* (autoimmune β-cell destruction → complete insulin deficiency)
- *Type 2 diabetes* (due to insulin resistance)
- *Gestational diabetes mellitus* (diabetes diagnosed in second/third trimester)
- *Specific types:* Endocrinopathies, drug/chemical induced, infections, and immune-mediated

RISK FACTORS

- First-degree relative diabetic
- High-risk ethnicity
- Obese [body mass index (BMI) >25, >23 for Asians]
- History of gestational diabetes
- Previous large baby (>4 kg)
- Bad obstetric history
- Unexplained stillbirth
- Congenitally malformed baby
- Persistent glycosuria
- Women with polycystic ovary syndrome (PCOS)
- Glycated hemoglobin (HbA1C) ≥5.7%

MATERNAL AND NEONATAL COMPLICATIONS IN DIABETIC PREGNANCIES

- *Antenatal complications:* Abortion, recurrent infection, hypertension, preeclampsia, polyhydramnios, malpresentations, premature labor, macrosomia, congenital malformation, intrauterine fetal demise, and stillbirth
- *Intrapartum complications:* Shoulder dystocia, birth injuries, instrumental delivery, and cesarean section (CS) prolonged labor, obstructed labor, uterine atony, postpartum hemorrhage
- *Neonatal:* Hypoglycemia, hyperbilirubinemia, respiratory distress, hypocalcemia, polycythemia hypomagnesemia, and neurodevelopmental abnormalities.

SCREENING AND DIAGNOSTIC CRITERIA

*Testing for GDM recommended **twice** during antenatal care (ANC):*

- *First testing:* At first antenatal contact
- *Second testing:* During 24–28 weeks of pregnancy (if the first test is negative)

Diabetes in Pregnancy Study Group of India Method

Single step method:

- Give 75 g oral glucose dissolved in 300 mL of water and blood sugar is measured after 2 hours of ingestion.
- Blood sugar level of ≥140 mg/dL is taken as cut off for diagnosis of GDM.

Oral Glucose Tolerance Test

Generally the diagnostic test of choice:

- It is done at the first antenatal visit and between 24 and 28 weeks of gestation.
- According to NICE, GDM diagnosed if any one of the following cut-offs is met, that is:
    - Fasting ≥100 mg/dL (≥5.6 mmol/L)
    - 1 first hour ≥180 mg/dL (≥10 mmol/L)
    - 2 hours ≥140 mg/dL (≥7.8 mmol/L)

MANAGEMENT

- According to FOGSI, any woman testing positive for GDM should start with medical nutrition therapy (MNT) and physical exercise for 2 weeks.
- Woman should walk/moderate aerobic exercise for 30 min/day (150 min/week).

- If GDM is not controlled with MNT (lifestyle changes), Insulin or Metformin is added along with MNT and physical exercise.

Medical Nutrition Therapy

Around 80–90% women with GDM can be managed by dietary restriction and do not require additional pharmacotherapy. Caloric restriction reduces the insulin resistance and brings down the blood sugar levels as a result.

- Recommended caloric intake is based on the pre-pregnancy body weight:
  - 35–40 kcal/kg/day for underweight (BMI <19 kg/m^2)
  - 30 kcal/kg/day for normal weight (19–24.9 kg/m^2)
  - 25 kcal/kg/day for overweight (BMI 25–29.9 kg/m^2)
  - 20 kcal/kg/day for obese (BMI ≥30 kg/m^2)
  - 12 kcal/kg/day for morbidly obese (BMI ≥40 kg/m^2)
- The total calories should be contributed by about 35–40% from carbohydrates, 20% from protein and 30–40% from fats with 10% from saturated fats.
- The distribution is usually into three main meals and three snacks.
- Complex carbohydrates such as whole-grain cereals preferred over simple carbohydrates.
- Sources of protein such as milk and milk products, fish, egg, chicken, pulses (dal), nuts, and green leafy vegetables must be advised.
- Diet containing high fiber (soluble fiber) is advised, e.g., flax seed, psyllium husk, oat bran, legumes, pectin, and root vegetables must be included in diet.
- Regarding exercise, 15–30 minutes of brisk walking after meal improves glycemic control.

Flowchart 1 displays how to approach a case of GDM.

Medical Management

- Metformin or insulin therapy added when blood sugar not controlled on MNT.
- Insulin is first drug of choice for GDM, Metformin can be given >20 weeks of gestation.
- Insulin is started if fasting blood sugar (FBS) >126 mg/dL or 2 hours PPBS >200 mg/dL any time during pregnancy along with MNT.

Metformin

- *Dosage:* 500 mg twice daily orally up to a maximum of 2 g/day
- If the woman's blood sugar is not controlled with the maximum dose of Metformin (2 g/day) and MNT, insulin is to be added.
- Hypoglycemia and weight gain with Metformin are less in comparison to insulin.
- Common side-effects with Metformin include diarrhea, nausea, stomach pain, heartburn, gastritis,

Flowchart 1: Diagnosis and management of GDM technical and operational guidelines.

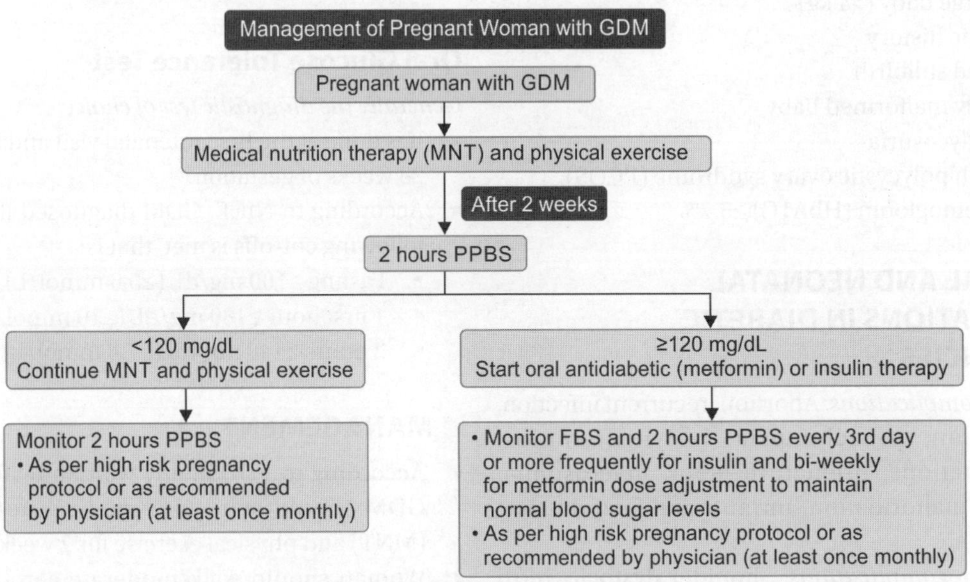

(FBS: fasting blood sugar; GDM: gestational diabetes mellitus; PPBS: postprandial blood sugar)
Source: Maternal Health Division, Ministry of Health and Family Welfare of India

and serious side effects are lactic acidosis and low blood sugar.

Insulin

Types of insulin:
- Rapid-acting insulin analogs—Lispro and Aspart
- Long-acting insulin analogs—Lantus
- Short-acting human insulin—Regular insulin
- Intermediate-acting insulin—Neutral Protamine Hagedorn (NPH) (isophane)

Site of insulin injection: Front/Lateral aspect of thigh or over abdomen, given subcutaneously only.

Insulin dosage in pregnancy: Total insulin required in different trimesters:
- *First trimester:* 0.7 U/kg
- *Second trimester:* 0.8 U/kg
- *Third trimester:* 0.9–1 U/kg

Dose of insulin calculated according to blood sugar level.

Insulin regimens: Most common regime is the four times daily injections:
- Three injections of regular short-acting insulin with three major meals plus bedtime injection of intermediate-acting insulin (NPH)
- Premeal insulin dose can be increased (~2 units at a time) depending on corresponding post-meal value, and NPH is increased if fasting glucose is high.

Another regimen of insulin therapy: "Twice daily regimen":
- A combination of regular and NPH insulin is used.
- The total dose calculated is divided into two, two-thirds of the total insulin dose given in the morning before breakfast, and one-third in the evening before dinner.
- The morning dose is constituted by two-thirds NPH and one-third regular or rapid-acting insulin, whereas the evening dose contains half NPH and half regular insulin.

Monitoring of blood sugar: The target values are as follows:
- Fasting <95 mg/dL
- *Postmeals:* 1 hour: <140 mg/dL, 2 hours: <120 mg/dL
- Fasting, premeal, 1-hour postmeal and bedtime blood sugar daily till target value
- Hypoglycemia is diagnosed when blood sugar level is <70 mg/dL
- It is important to recognize symptoms of hypoglycemia and treat immediately.

Hypoglycemia Early Symptoms

Hypoglycemia early symptoms include hand tremors, sweating, palpitations, hunger, easy fatigability, headache, mood changes, irritability, low attentiveness, and tingling sensation around mouth/lips.

Severe Symptoms

Severe symptoms include confusion, abnormal behavior or both, visual disturbances, nervousness, or anxiety. *Uncommon*—seizures and loss of consciousness.

Preconception Care

Women with diabetes planning for pregnancy should have HbA1c <48 mmol/mol (6.5%) and Folic acid 5 mg/day, 1 month prior to conception till 12 weeks of pregnancy to ↓risk of neural tube defect (NTD) in baby.

Antenatal Care

High-risk pregnancy, multidisciplinary team in joint consultation with diabetologist, monitored for hypertension in pregnancy, proteinuria and other obstetric complications.

Increased risk for IUFD, strict and regular fetal surveillance needed:
- Fetal heart monitored by auscultation on each antenatal visit.
- Pregnant women enquired about daily fetal movement count.
- <20 weeks of pregnancy, a targeted anomaly scan USG at 18–20 weeks.
- Fetal growth assessment (fetal biometry and amniotic fluid) performed at 28–30 weeks gestation and repeated at 34–36 weeks of gestation.

LABOR AND DELIVERY

- Pregnant women with GDM with good control of blood sugar (2-hour PPBS levels <120 mg/dL) may be delivered at their respective health facility.
- Pregnant women with GDM on insulin therapy with uncontrolled blood sugar should deliver at higher center.

Timing of Delivery

- Patients with gestational diabetes well controlled on diet can be followed till 40 weeks.

TABLE 1: Regime of insulin infusion.

Blood sugar level (mg/dL)	*Amount of insulin added in 500 mL of normal saline*	*Rate of normal saline infusion*
90–120	0	100 mL/h (16 drops/min)
120–140	4 U	100 mL/h (16 drops/min)
140–180	6 U	100 mL/h (16 drops/min)
180	8 U	100 mL/h (16 drops/min)

- Delivery <39 weeks is not advised as GDM associated with delay in lung maturity of the fetus.
- If well-controlled GDM not delivered, induction of labor (IOL) considered ≥39 weeks.
- Those on insulin, IOL at 38 weeks reduces incidence of macrosomia and shoulder dystocia.
- If associated with complications—PIH or BOH should deliver at 37–38^{+6} weeks, but if associated with abnormal antepartum fetal tests/failed glycemic control should deliver at late preterm 34–36^{+6} weeks.
- Vaginal delivery is mode of delivery, cesarean section (CS) for obstetric indications only.
- In case of fetal macrosomia (EFBW >4.5 kg), elective lower segment caesarean section (LSCS) at 39 weeks.

During Labor

Women with GDM on medical management require blood sugar monitoring by glucometer.

- Morning dose of insulin/Metformin is omitted on the day of induction/labor and should be started with 1–2 hourly monitoring of blood sugar.
- Intravenous (IV) infusion with Normal Saline (NS) and regular insulin according to blood sugar.

Table 1 shows the dose and rate of IV Insulin according to blood sugar level.

Postdelivery Follow-up

Early breastfeeding along with immediate newborn care to prevent hypoglycemia.

Cut off capillary blood glucose for hypoglycemia in normal birth weight newborn is <45 mg/dL and <54 mg/dL in case of intrauterine growth restriction (IUGR), done at 1–2 hours of birth.

- These women are at high risk to develop type 2 diabetes mellitus in future.
- Maternal glucose levels usually return to normal after delivery.
- 75 g oral glucose tolerance test (OGTT) (fasting and 2-hour PP) 4–6 weeks postpartum, then annually.

Contraception

- Diabetics can be offered all contraceptive choices that are available to non-diabetics.
- Long-acting reversible contraception with Cu-T/ Levonorgestrel intrauterine system (LNG-IUS) or progestin implants provide most effective contraception and should be recommended.
- Low-dose COCP prescribed to diabetics without vasculopathy and who do not smoke; instead, Progestogen-only pill (POP) can be prescribed to women with vascular disease.
- WHO advises unrestricted use of Cu-T intrauterine contraceptive device (IUCD) in all types of diabetics.

SUGGESTED READING

1. ACOG Practice Bulletin PB Number 190: Gestational Diabetes Mellitus. Obstet Gynecol. 2018;131(2):e49-e64.
2. ACOG Clinical Practice Update: Screening for Gestational and Pregestational Diabetes in Pregnancy and Postpartum. Obstetr Gynecol. 2024;144(1):e20-3.
3. Maternal Health Division, Ministry of Health and Family Welfare of India. (2018). Diagnosis and management of Gestational Diabetes Mellitus Technical and Operational Guidelines. [online] Available from https://nhm.gov.in/New_Updates_2018/NHM_Components/RMNCH_MH_Guidelines/Gestational-Diabetes-Mellitus.pdf [Last accessed September, 2024].
4. Mishra R. Ian Donald obstetrics, 9th edition. India: Wolters Kluwer; 2020.
5. NICE. (2015). Diabetes in pregnancy: Management from preconception to the postnatal period NICE guideline [NG3]. [online] Available from https://www.nice.org.uk/guidance/ng3/chapter/recommendations [Last accessed September, 2024].
6. Singh R, Rajorhia A, Jaipuriar AS. (2018). Gestational Diabetes. [online] Available from https://www.fogsi.org/wp-content/uploads/committee-2020-activities/vol-17-endocrinology-committee-newsletter.pdf [Last accessed September, 2024].
7. Treatment of diabetes by obesity management: ADA Guideline (Published On 4 Jan 2021).

CHAPTER 27

Thyroid Disorders in Pregnancy

INTRODUCTION

Thyroid disorder is second most common endocrine condition affecting women of reproductive age (first is diabetes). Trimester-specific thyroid-stimulating hormone (TSH) reference ranges—first trimester 0.1–2.5 mU/L, second trimester 0.2–3 mU/L, third trimester 0.3–3 mU/L. Universal screening for hypothyroidism for all antenatal women, especially in the first trimester, should be preferred over targeted case-based screening.

RISK FACTORS FOR THYROID DYSFUNCTION

- History of thyroid dysfunction/thyroid surgery
- Family history of thyroid disease
- Goiter
- Positive thyroid autoantibodies
- Clinical signs/symptoms of hypothyroidism
- Type 1 diabetes
- Autoimmune disease
- History of subfertility
- History of miscarriage/preterm labor
- History of therapeutic head or neck irradiation
- Age >30 years
- History of treatment with Amiodarone/Lithium
- Recent exposure to iodinated radiological contrast agents

EFFECTS OF PREGNANCY ON THYROID

- ↑Serum β-human chorionic gonadotropin (hCG) (α-subunit closely related structurally to serum TSH) (peaks at 8–10 weeks,) stimulates TSH receptors to release thyroid hormone and suppress ↓serum TSH level → gestational hyperthyroidism (1–3% of all pregnancies).
- Due to ↑estrogen, ↑ thyroxine-binding globulin (TBG) synthesis (reaches twice the nonpregnant level by 16–20 weeks) and ↓clearance → goitrogenic effect, i.e.,↑ total T3 and T4, though free hormone level is unchanged.
- Due to ↑ glomerular filtration rate (GFR) and plasma clearance, renal excretion of iodine increases, as well as to meet fetal demand, requirement of iodine for synthesis of thyroid hormone increases.
- Concentration of deiodinase III (converts T4 to active T3) increases in the placenta with gestation, releasing iodine where it is required for transport to the fetus.

EFFECTS OF THYROID ON PREGNANCY

Hypothyroidism in Pregnancy

Overt—0.5%, subclinical—2.5%. As fetus requires maternal thyroxine T4 till 12–14 weeks gestation (due to fetal thyroid immaturity), neurodevelopmental delay is a risk for infants.

Complications of hypothyroidism in pregnancy:

- *Maternal:* Spontaneous abortion, pregnancy-induced hypertension (PIH), anemia, postpartum hemorrhage (PPH), cardiac dysfunction, preeclampsia, abruptio placentae, and preterm labor
- *Fetal and neonatal:* Prematurity, low birth weight (LBW), fetal distress in labor, congenital malformation, stillbirth, perinatal death, neurodevelopmental delay, and congenital hypothyroidism (autoimmune)
- *Prepregnancy assessment:* If known hypothyroid, thyroxine dose should be adjusted to maintain serum TSH <2.5 mU/L prior to pregnancy. Women with risk factors like autoimmune diseases should be screened with serum TSH.
- *Antenatal (prenatal) management*—since fetus is entirely dependent on mother for its thyroxine supply during first trimester and later for iodine, thyroxine and iodine should be supplemented from early pregnancy to those who are hypothyroid/likely to be iodine deficient. If already on thyroxine, dose should be increased by 30% (25 µg) as soon as pregnancy is diagnosed and then titrated by TSH levels. If hypothyroidism detected first time during pregnancy, Levothyroxine should be started at 2 µg/kg/day and titrated according to serum TSH level after 4 weeks.

Flowchart 1: Approach to hypothyroidism in pregnancy.

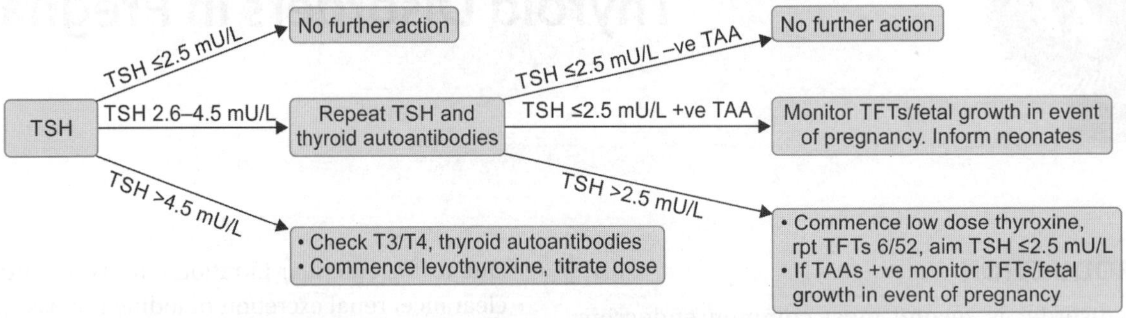

(TAA: thyroid autoantibody; TFT: thyroid function test; TSH: thyroid-stimulating hormone)

Therapy should be monitored by TSH levels every 6–8 weeks throughout pregnancy. According to a TOG article, following approach **(Flowchart 1)** is suggested.

Iron/calcium supplements, if prescribed to pregnant women, should be advised to be consumed at least 4 hours after LT4 dose.

- *Postnatal:* For subclinical hypothyroidism or if LT4 dose ≤50 µg/day, postpartum thyroxine treatment can be discontinued (if started in pregnancy) and thyroid function test (TFT) repeated 6 weeks after delivery/sooner if symptomatic. For overt hypothyroidism, thyroxine dose should be reduced to prepregnancy level immediately after delivery and TFT repeated at 6 weeks.

Neonatal assessment should be done after 5–10 days of delivery.

Hyperthyroidism in Pregnancy

A medical history, physical examination, and testing of the maternal blood FT4 or TT4 concentrations should be performed when a suppressed serum TSH is found in the first trimester (a serum TSH below 0.1 mU/L in some cases, even undetectable) by week 11. Serum total T4 and T3 levels >1.5 times the nonpregnant range should be used to diagnose thyrotoxicosis in the second and third trimesters of pregnancy. Causes are Grave's disease (90% cases—↑fT4 + TSH receptor antibodies), multinodular goiter, toxic adenoma, thyroiditis, carcinoma, and drug-induced amiodarone.

- Incidence—0.1–0.2%
- *Gestational transient hyperthyroidism*—molar pregnancy, multiple pregnancy, and hyperemesis gravidarum (due to excessive production of β-hCG hormone). No specific treatment required, and it resolves spontaneously as hCG level falls.
- *Maternal complications*—preterm labor, preeclampsia, fetal growth restriction (FGR), thyroid storm, congestive cardiac failure, and even death
- *Fetal*—LBW babies, neonatal thyrotoxicosis, and perinatal mortality
  - H/O—palpitations, tachycardia, heat intolerance, fatigue, diplopia, and photophobia
  - O/E—swelling in thyroid area which moves with deglutition (diffuse/nodular)
- *Investigations*: TFT (T4 and TSH), thyroid antibodies [TSH receptor, thyroid stimulating Ab, and thyroid peroxidase (TPO) Ab], ultrasonography (USG), and fine needle aspiration cytology (FNAC). Fetal thyroid size by periodic USG after 20 weeks, and cordocentesis for fetal thyroid hormones if scan suggestive of fetal goiter, FGR or hydrops
- *Course of Grave's disease during pregnancy*—due to natural immunosuppressive effect of pregnancy, it tends to remit with advancing gestation and relapse postpartum, thus dose of antithyroid medication may be lessened during second and third trimester. Also, in early fetal goiter, the dosage of antithyroid drug (ATD) should be decreased or discontinued in the mother. Intraamniotic LT4 instillation can be done after confirmation of fetal hypothyroidism.
- *Treatment:* Propylthiouracil (PTU) preferred as it blocks synthesis of T4 and T3, inhibits peripheral conversion of T4 to T3, and also causes immune-suppression. FT4 and TSH monitored every 2–8 weeks. Side effects include skin rash, hepatotoxicity, and agranulocytosis. As it is not associated with congenital malformation, guidelines recommend its use in first trimester and switch over to Carbimazole in second trimester due to concern of side effects. Methimazole found to be associated with aplasia cutis congenita (scalp defects),

esophageal atresia with tracheoesophageal fistula (TOF), and choanal atresia.

- Beta-blockers (Propranolol) recommended only for the symptomatic control of thyrotoxicosis or while awaiting response to the antithyroid medications or surgery.
- Surgery—total thyroidectomy preferred over subtotal due to high risk of recurrence, best done in second trimester (radioactive iodine CI and pregnancy avoided at least for 6 months after).

- *Postnatal*—breastfeeding safe with PTU, minimum amount excreted in breast milk as compared to Carbimazole/Methimazole (dose should be divided and breastfeed baby before taking medicine)
- *Neonatal assessment:* Close monitoring required as transient thyrotoxicosis may occur in NB >7–10 days due to presence of circulating maternal autoantibodies as antithyroid medication gets cleared from fetal plasma—vomiting, diarrhea, dehydration, weight loss, irritability, and poor feeding. Symptomatic and supportive treatment till (4–6 weeks) maternal antibodies are cleared. 15% mortality if untreated.

POSTPARTUM THYROIDITIS (PPT)

Subacute destructive autoimmune condition during first postpartum year, with no prior history of thyroid disease, resulting in either transient or permanent thyroid dysfunction. It comprises thyrotoxicosis followed by hypothyroidism; while one-third of patients may manifest both phases, the others may be either only thyrotoxic or hypothyroid. The thyrotoxic phase of postpartum thyroiditis (PPT) is usually asymptomatic (symptoms, e.g., palpitations, weariness, and irritability), whereas the hypothyroid phase of PPT can cause symptoms such as paresthesia, dry skin, tiredness, and cold intolerance.

Three clinical manifestations of PPT—(1) transient hyperthyroidism (32%), (2) transient hypothyroidism (43%), and (3) transient hyperthyroidism followed by hypothyroidism and then recovery, which is the classic form of PPT (25%). Hyperthyroidism occurs between 1 to 3 months after delivery and hypothyroidism at 3–8 months, finally euthyroidism by 1 year. **Flowchart 2** displays approach to different phases of PPT.

Symptoms, presence, or absence of thyrotropin receptor antibodies and T4:T3 ratio can help distinguish

Flowchart 2: Different phases of postpartum thyroiditis (PPT).

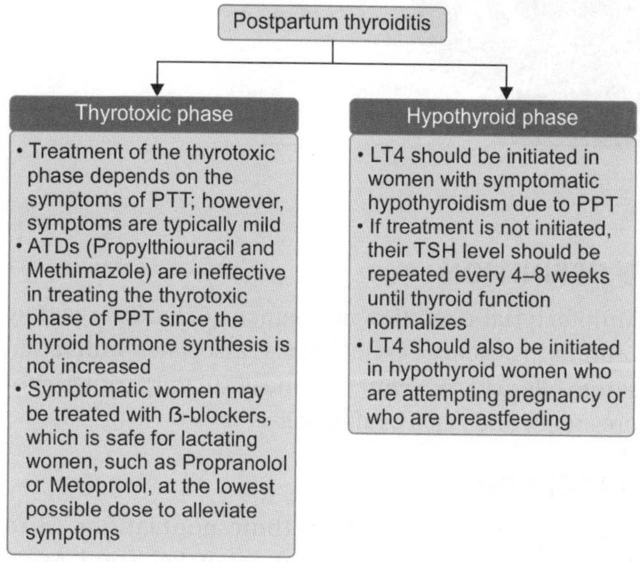

(ATD: antithyroid drug; PTT: partial thromboplastin time; TSH: thyroid-stimulating hormone)

PPT from Graves' disease (GD) or other thyrotoxicosis conditions.

Treatment

For hyperthyroidism symptomatic treatment with beta-blockers. ATDs are not recommended for the treatment of the thyrotoxic phase of PPT. Following the resolution of the thyrotoxic phase of PPT, serum TSH should be measured in approximately 4–8 weeks (or if new symptoms develop) to screen for the hypothyroid phase.

LT4 should be considered in women who have symptomatic PPT-induced hypothyroidism or TSH >10 mU/L. Their TSH level should be assessed every 4–8 weeks until thyroid function is normalized if no therapy is initiated. Additionally, hypothyroid women who are planning a pregnancy or who are breastfeeding should begin taking LT4. If LT4 is initiated for PPT, discontinuation of therapy should be attempted after 12 months.

Women with a prior history of PPT should have TSH testing annually to evaluate the development of permanent hypothyroidism.

SUGGESTED READING

1. Girling J. Thyroid disease in pregnancy. Obstetr Gynaecol. 2008;10:237-43.
2. Indian Thyroid Society & FOGSI Joint Recommendations on Thyroid disorders in Pregnancy, 2019.

CHAPTER 28

Cholestasis in Pregnancy

DEFINITION

Multifactorial condition of pregnancy characterized by pruritus in absence of skin diseases associated with raised serum bile acid concentration, mostly in third trimester of pregnancy and resolves after delivery.

INCIDENCE

7/1,000 in women of multiethnic populations, ↑ to 12–15/1,000 women of Indian-Asian/Pakistani-Asian origin.

According to recent RCOG Guideline (symptoms + nonfasting serum bile acid level):

- Gestational pruritus → itching + peak bile acid concentrations <19 μmol/L
- Mild intrahepatic cholestasis of pregnancy (IHCP) → itching + raised peak bile acid concentrations 19–39 μmol/L
- Moderate IHCP → itching + raised peak bile acid concentrations 40–99 μmol/L
- Severe IHCP → itching + raised peak bile acid concentrations ≥100 μmol/L

RISK FACTORS

- Past obstetric history of IHCP, multiple pregnancy, chronic hepatitis C virus (HCV) infection, advanced maternal age, genetic susceptibility (↑ risk in first-degree relatives/ethnic groups), role of ↑ estrogen (most common in second half of pregnancy, multiple pregnancy, and resolves after delivery), environmental factors (associated with Selenium deficient diet, vitamin D deficiency), underlying liver disease (chronic liver disease/nonalcoholic cirrhosis)
- *Structured history*—pruritus starts at palms and soles, worse at night, generalized may be associated with right upper quadrant pain, nausea, poor appetite, steatorrheas, and sleep disturbances.

CLINICAL EXAMINATION

Scratch marks/excoriations/prurigo nodules secondary to itching but no primary skin lesion, done to rule out other causes, i.e., *differential diagnosis:*

- Pregnancy-specific causes of pruritus—pruritus gravidarum, atopic eruption of pregnancy, polymorphic eruption of pregnancy, pemphigoid gestationis, and prurigo/pruritus folliculitis of pregnancy
- Preexisting skin causes—atopic dermatitis, allergic or drug reaction, and systemic disease such as liver, renal, and thyroid disease
- Pregnancy-specific causes of deranged liver function tests-acute fatty liver of pregnancy (AFLP), hemolysis, elevated liver enzymes, and low platelet count (HELLP), preeclampsia (PE), and hyperemesis gravidarum
- Preexisting causes of deranged LFT—viral hepatitis, primary biliary cirrhosis, primary sclerosing cholangitis, autoimmune hepatitis, biliary obstruction, and veno-occlusive disease.

DIAGNOSIS

If on history and clinical examination, no other cause such as infection, autoimmune, or structural, is suspected then no further investigation is required (as thought previously that it is a diagnosis of exclusion, after going through various blood tests and USG). Additional investigation required only when *atypical* features—markedly elevated transaminases, early-onset IHCP in first/second trimester, a rapidly progressive biochemical picture, sign/symptom of liver failure or acute infection, or if does not normalize 4 weeks after birth; and referred to hepatologist.

- *Effects on mother:* Itching more at night, may interfere with sleep, thus affecting mental health. ↑ Chance of preeclampsia and gestational diabetes mellitus (GDM), hepatitis, hepatobiliary disease/gallbladder (GB) stone and rarely dark urine, pale stools, and jaundice.

- *Effects on fetus:* ↑ chance of meconium-stained liquor (MSL), preterm birth (spontaneous/induced), ↑ respiratory distress syndrome (RDS) and neonatal intensive care unit (NICU) admission, and stillborn (more associated with severe type with bile acid ≥100 μmol/L). Cause of sudden fetal demise is cardiac arrhythmia due to anoxia or spasm of placental blood vessels; ↑ risk in severe IHCP (SBA >100 μmol/L) and/or associated with comorbidities (GDM/PE/multiple pregnancy).

MANAGEMENT

High-risk pregnancy (HRP). Consultant-led unit, screening for GDM by diabetes in pregnancy study group of India (DIPSI), frequent monitoring of BP + protein in urine in each antenatal visit to rule out PE. For women with IHCP (pruritus + ↑SBA) repeat LFT and SBA after 1 week to confirm the diagnosis and degree of severity as well as nature of progression and subsequent frequency of biochemical assessment:

- Mild IHCP (15–40 μmol/L) → fortnightly till 38 weeks, then weekly and plan delivery at 40 weeks
- Moderate IHCP (40–99 μmol/L) → weekly from 35 weeks and plan delivery at 38–39 weeks
- Severe IHCP (≥100 μmol/L) → no further testing, plan delivery (RCOG 35–36 weeks) [Society for Maternal-Fetal Medicine (SMFM) 36 weeks]. SMFM recommends steroids for fetal lung maturity if delivering <37 weeks. Sometimes preterm delivery <36 weeks if excruciating and unremitting maternal pruritus not relieved with medication, deranged LFT, O/H of intrauterine demise (IUD) <36 weeks due to IHCP.

Fetal monitoring—as **no FGR**, so no role of routine USG/color Doppler/biophysical profile (BPP)/cardiotocography (CTG) (neither predict nor prevent stillborn); but woman is asked to monitor the quantity and quality of fetal movement daily and report immediately if there is any change in it. During labor, especially in severe type IHCP, presence of MSL, or risk factors such as GDM, PE, and multiple pregnancy, CEFM should be done.

DRUG TREATMENT

To reduce itching—topical emollient, antihistamines (Chlorpheniramine—sedation) at bedtime. Ursodeoxycholic acid (UDCA)—first-line agents for treatment of maternal symptoms, 10–15 mg/kg/day in divided doses (side effects—nausea and dizziness), if pruritus not relieved within 2 weeks, dose increased every 1–2 weeks to maximum dose of 21 mg/kg/day. Small improvement in itch score and alanine aminotransferase (ALT) level, but fetal, and neonatal outcome not improved. Vitamin K (Menadiol Sodium Phosphate at a dose of 10 mg daily) only if steatorrhea and/or abnormal PT.

FOLLOW-UP

Repeat SBA and LFT after 4 weeks of delivery. If itching and/or abnormal LFT/SBA persists 6 weeks after delivery, then refer to hepatologist.

CONTRACEPTION

All hormonal preparation including combined hormonal contraception (CHC) can be given if there is no history of contraception-induced cholestasis, and PGN-only or non-hormonal method if history of hormone (OGN)-induced cholestasis. If on COC, regular follow-up with LFT every 3–6 month. Similarly, no CI to HRT in menopausal women if no history of hormone-induced cholestasis.

FUTURE PREGNANCIES

As chance of recurrence is high (60–70%), baseline LFT and SBA should be done along with booking blood investigations.

SUGGESTED READING

1. Girling J, Knight CL, Chappell L; Royal College of Obstetricians and Gynaecologists. Intrahepatic cholestasis of pregnancy: Green-top Guideline No. 43. BJOG. 2022; 129(13):e95-e114.
2. Society for Maternal-Fetal Medicine (SMFM); Lee RH, Mara Greenberg, Metz TD, Pettker CM. Society for Maternal-Fetal Medicine Consult Series #53: Intrahepatic cholestasis of pregnancy: Replaces Consult #13, April 2011. Am J Obstet Gynecol. 2021;224(2):B2-B9.

CHAPTER 29

Human Immunodeficiency Virus in Pregnancy

INTRODUCTION

Antenatal human immunodeficiency virus (HIV) care by a multidisciplinary team (MDT), and perinatal mental health assessment especially for depression should be done at booking, 4–6 weeks postpartum and 3–4 months postpartum. Sexual health screening should be done in pregnant women newly diagnosed with HIV and genital tract infections should be treated.

LABORATORY TESTING

No additional baseline investigations required as compared to nonpregnant women with HIV, i.e., HIV resistance testing (<28 weeks) before starting antiretroviral therapy (ART), CD4 cell count at baseline and at delivery; HIV viral load at 2–4 weeks after commencing combination ART (cART), at least once every trimester, at 36 weeks and at delivery; liver function tests (LFTs) should be performed before initiation of cART and then with each routine blood test.

ANTIRETROVIRAL THERAPY USE IN PREGNANCY

All women not on cART should commence cART:

- In second trimester with baseline viral load ≤30,000 HIV RNA copies/mL
- At start of second trimester, or as soon as possible, in women with baseline viral load of 30,000–100,000 HIV RNA copies/mL
- Within first trimester if viral load >100,000 HIV RNA copies/mL and/or CD4 cell count <200 cells/mm^3. All women should have commenced cART by week 24 of pregnancy. Start Tenofovir/Abacavir with Emtricitabine/Lamivudine and third agent in cART should be Efavirenz/Atazanavir. Zidovudine monotherapy is not recommended and should only be used in women declining cART with a viral load of <10,000 HIV RNA copies/mL and willing to have a cesarean section.

Table 1 shows the dosage schedule and common side effects of ART drugs and **Table 2** displays clinical and laboratory monitoring of patients on ART.

DYNAMICS OF PERINATAL TRANSMISSION

Mother-to-child transmission (MTCT) is the most common cause of pediatric HIV infection. The risk of transmission to the fetus can be categorized based on the timing of transmission.

- *In utero (5–6%):* By transplacental passage
- *Intrapartum (13–18%):* By maternal-fetal transfusion and contact of fetal skin and mucous membrane with maternal secretions during delivery
- *Postpartum (12–14%):* During early weeks of breast-feeding.

TABLE 1: Commonly used antiretroviral therapy (ART) medications.

Name of antiretroviral (ARV)	*Dose*	*Major side-effects*
Tenofovir disoproxil fumarate (TDF)	300 mg once daily	Nephrotoxicity, hypophosphatemia
Lamivudine (3TC)	300 mg once daily	*Very few side effects:* Hypersensitivity, rarely pancreatitis
Efavirenz (EFV)	600 mg once daily	Neuropsychiatric symptoms such as hallucinations, suicidal ideations, nightmares, and vivid dreams
Lopinavir/ritonavir (LPV/r)	400/100 mg twice daily (dose of FDC tablet of LPV (200 mg)/ritonavir (50 mg)—two tablets BD)	Gastrointestinal disturbances, glucose intolerance, lipodystrophy, and hyperlipidemia

TABLE 2: Laboratory monitoring of pregnant women receiving antiretroviral therapy.

Assessment	*Baseline*	*2 weeks*	*4 weeks*	*8 weeks*	*12 weeks*	*Every 6 months*	*Comment*
Clinical evaluation	✓	✓	✓	✓	✓	✓	Every month
Adherence counseling	✓	✓	✓	✓	✓	✓	Every month
Weight	✓	✓	✓	✓	✓	✓	Every month
Hemoglobin	✓	✓	✓	–	✓	✓	
LFT	✓		–	–	–	✓	As and when required clinically
Urinalysis	✓	–	–	–	–	✓	Specifically for TDF-based regimen)

(LFT: liver function test; TDF: Tenofovir Disoproxil Fumarate)

Flowchart 1: Displaying four goals of PPTCT.

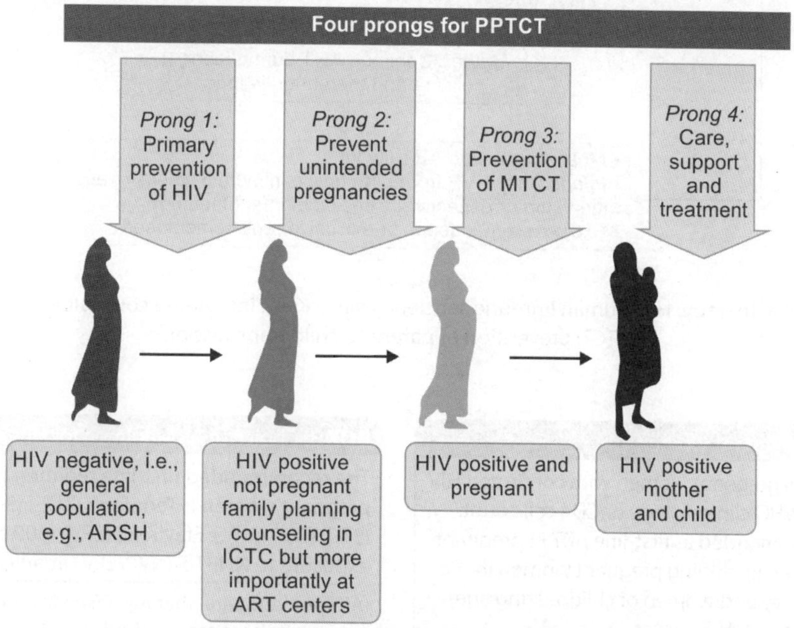

(ARSH: Adolescent Reproductive and Sexual Health; ART: antiretroviral therapy; HIV: human immunodeficiency virus; ICTC: integrated counseling and testing center; MTCT: mother-to-child transmission; PPTCT: prevention of parent to child transmission)

PREVENTION OF PARENT-TO-CHILD TRANSMISSION OF HIV USING MULTIDRUG ANTIRETROVIRAL REGIMEN IN INDIA

Goals of the Parent-to-Child Transmission Program (Flowcharts 1 and 2)

- *Prong 1:* Primary prevention of HIV, especially among women of childbearing age
- *Prong 2:* Preventing unintended pregnancies among women living with HIV
- *Prong 3:* Prevent HIV transmission from pregnant women infected with HIV to their child
- *Prong 4:* Provide care, support, and treatment to women living with HIV, her children and family in women in childbearing age.

CRITERIA FOR ART INITIATION

In HIV-infected pregnant women, the dictum should be "do not delay ART initiation". The eligibility criteria for initiating ART in HIV-positive pregnant women are shown in **Box 1**

Indications for Cotrimoxazole prophylactic therapy (CPT) in pregnancy are shown in **Box 2**.

Flowchart 2: Summary of technical guidelines and options for the more efficacious PPTCT regimen.

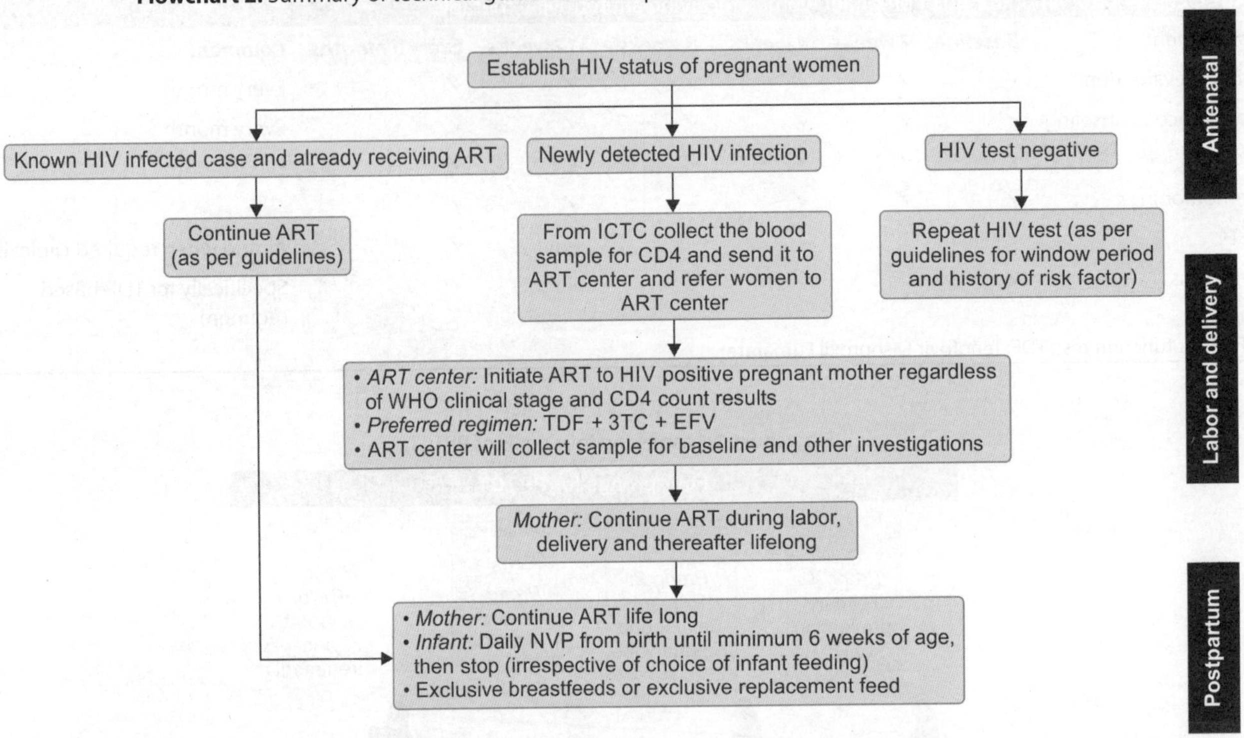

(ART: antiretroviral therapy; HIV: human immunodeficiency virus; ICTC: integrated counseling and testing center; PPTCT: prevention of parent to child transmission)

BOX 1: ART eligibility in pregnant women.

- Initiate lifelong ART in all pregnant women with confirmed HIV infection regardless of WHO clinical stage or CD4 cell count. TDF + 3TC + EFV is recommended as first-line ART in pregnant and breastfeeding women (including pregnant women in the first trimester of pregnancy and women of childbearing age)
- ART shall be initiated only at ART center

(ART: antiretroviral therapy; EFV: efavirenz; TDF: Tenofovir Disoproxil Fumarate)

BOX 2: Starting cotrimoxazole in pregnancy.

- Cotrimoxazole should be started if CD4 count is ≤250 cells/mm^3 and continued through pregnancy, delivery, and breastfeeding as per national guidelines (*Dose:* Double strength tablet–1 tablet daily)
- Ensure that pregnant women take their folate supplements regularly

PRINCIPLES OF MANAGEMENT

All HIV-infected pregnant women should start ART:

- Start ART as soon as possible and continue ART throughout pregnancy, delivery, breastfeeding period, and thereafter lifelong.

BOX 3: Choice of ART regimen for HIV-infected pregnant women.

The recommended first-line regimen for HIV-infected pregnant women is Tenofovir (TDF) (300 mg) + Lamuvidine (3TC) (300 mg) + Efavirenz (EFV) (600 mg) (if there is no prior exposure to NNRTIS (NVP/EFV) at any gestational age

(ART: antiretroviral therapy; EFV: efavirenz; NNRTIS: non-nucleoside reverse transcriptase inhibitor; NVP: nevirapine; TDF: Tenofovir Disoproxil Fumarate)

- Even if the pregnant women present very late in pregnancy (including those who present after 36 weeks of gestation), ART should be initiated promptly.

Choice of ART Regimen for HIV-infected Pregnant Women (Box 3)

Box 4 shows recommended treatment for pregnant and lactating women and their infants.

OBSTETRIC MANAGEMENT

Antenatal Care

Apart from routine antenatal investigations, combined screening test for fetal aneuploidies and noninvasive

BOX 4: First-line ART for pregnant and breastfeeding women and ARV drugs for their infants.

- A once-daily fixed-dose combination of TDF + 3TC + EFV is recommended as first-line ART in pregnant and breastfeeding women, including pregnant women in the first trimester of pregnancy and women of childbearing age
- Infants of mothers who are receiving ART and are exclusively breastfeeding or doing exclusive replacement feeding should receive at least 6 weeks of infant prophylaxis with daily syrup Nevirapine. Infant prophylaxis should begin at birth or when HIV exposure is known

(ART: antiretroviral therapy; ARV: antiretroviral; EFV: efavirenz; TDF: Tenofovir Disoproxil Fumarate)

prenatal testing (NIPT) for those who screen as high risk is recommended as this will decrease need of invasive testing. Invasive prenatal diagnostic testing should not be performed until HIV status is known and should ideally be deferred until HIV viral load has been suppressed to <50 HIV RNA copies/mL. If not on cART and the invasive diagnostic test procedure cannot be delayed until viral suppression is achieved, it is recommended that women should commence cART to include Raltegravir and be given a single dose of Nevirapine (NVP) 2–4 hours prior to the procedure. External cephalic version (ECV) can be offered to women with plasma viral load <50 HIV RNA copies/mL.

Mode of Delivery

If on cART, a decision regarding mode of delivery should be made after plasma HIV viral load results at 36 weeks. If plasma viral load <50 HIV RNA copies/mL at 36 weeks (no obstetric contraindications), plan for vaginal delivery.

For viral load of 50–399 HIV RNA copies/mL at 36 weeks, prelabor CS (PLCS) should be **considered**. If viral load is ≥400 HIV RNA copies/mL at 36 weeks, PLCS is **recommended**. Vaginal birth after CS (VBAC) can be offered to women with a viral load <50 HIV RNA copies/mL. Where indication for CS is the prevention of vertical transmission, CS should be undertaken between 38 and 39 weeks of gestation.

Where PLCS is undertaken only for obstetric indications and plasma viral load is <50 HIV RNA copies/mL, the usual obstetric considerations apply and the CS will usually be performed after 39 weeks of gestation. Intrapartum intravenous Zidovudine infusion is recommended if viral load >1,000 HIV RNA copies/mL plasma who present in labor or with spontaneous rupture of membrane (SROM) or who are admitted for PLCS and considered between 50 and 1,000 HIV RNA copies/mL.

Algorithm for ART for pregnant women and their infants shown in **Flowchart 3**.

ANTIRETROVIRAL PROPHYLAXIS FOR INFANTS BORN TO MOTHERS RECEIVING LIFE-LONG ART

The infant antiretroviral (ARV) prophylaxis where mothers are receiving ART is daily NVP for 6 weeks (i.e., till the first immunization visit for the infant), regardless of whether

Flowchart 3: ART in pregnant and breastfeeding women, and their infants.

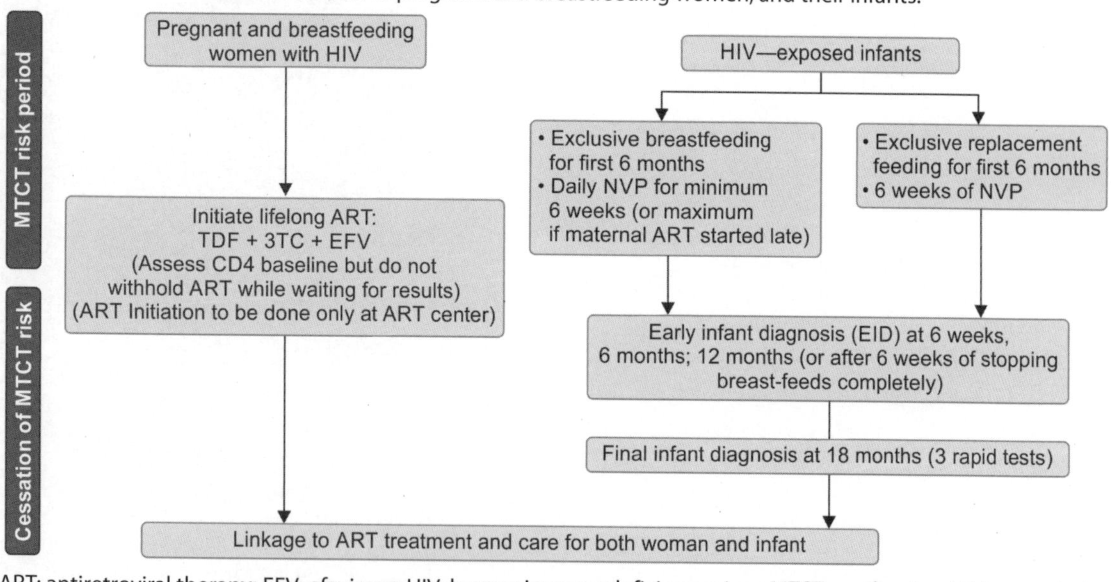

(ART: antiretroviral therapy; EFV: efavirenz; HIV: human immunodeficiency virus; MTCT: mother-to-child transmission; NVP: nevirapine; TDF: Tenofovir Disoproxil Fumarate)

the infant is exclusively breastfed or receives exclusive replacement feeding.

SUGGESTED READING

1. HIVA. (2018). British HIV Association guidelines for the management of HIV in pregnancy and postpartum 2018 (2020 third interim update). [online] Available from https://www.bhiva.org/file/5f1aab1ab9aba/BHIVA-Pregnancy-guidelines-2020-3rd-interim-update.pdf [Last accessed September, 2024].
2. NACO Guidelines. (2013). Prevention of Parent to Child Transmission (PPTCT) of HIV using Multi Drug Anti-Retroviral Regimen in India December, 2013. [online] Available from https://naco.gov.in/sites/default/files/National_Guidelines_for_PPTCT.pdf [Last accessed September, 2023].

CHAPTER 30

Syphilis in Pregnancy

INTRODUCTION

- Bacterial sexually transmitted infection (STI), caused by *Treponema pallidum*, a spirochaete, is the most common congenital infection worldwide. If a pregnant lady has syphilis, mother-to-fetus transmission can occur, ↑neonatal morbidity and mortality. Hence, its testing remains part of the antenatal screening program.
- Risk factors—low-socioeconomic status, multiparity, history of STIs, use of illicit drugs, multiple sexual partners, and poor antenatal care
- Transmission—sexual contact—genitally/extragenital (anal/rectal/oral), transplacental
- Stages—early (primary, secondary, and early latent) and late—late latent and tertiary
- Primary—Incubation period = 21 days (9–90)—**painless** single chancre at genitalia/multiple **painful** ulcers extragenital site, heals spontaneously in 3–8 weeks, 25% untreated→ secondary
- Secondary—4–10 weeks >initial chancre, mucocutaneous rash at palms and soles/flu-like symptoms, such as loss of appetite, lymphadenopathy, meningitis, eye disease (e.g., uveitis and optic neuropathy), hepatitis, glomerulonephritis, splenomegaly, and perianal condyloma lata. It resolves within 1–3 months, 30% of untreated → tertiary/late syphilis with cardiovascular and neurological manifestations.
- Vertical transmission—100% in primary, 40% in early latent and 10% in late latent stage of syphilis. From 14 weeks spirochete crosses placenta and causes fetal infection, increases as pregnancy progresses. In 30–40% intrauterine demise (IUD) occurs and of those who survive, around one-third will be born with signs of congenital syphilis.

FETAL AND NEONATAL INFECTION

Miscarriage, premature births, low birth weight babies, stillbirth, congenital syphilis, and neonatal mortality. Initially, placental infection followed by fetal hepatic dysfunction and amniotic fluid infection can lead to fetal growth restriction (FGR), hepatomegaly, hematological abnormalities (anemia, thrombocytopenia), ascites, and hydrops. Obstetric ultrasonography (USG) may show distorted fetal long bones or fetal hydrops, ascites, hepatosplenomegaly, intrahepatic calcifications, and placentomegaly.

DIAGNOSIS

- Direct *T. pallidum* demonstration in lesions/infected lymph nodes by dark ground microscopy or polymerase chain reaction (PCR).
- *Treponemal-specific antibody* tests include fluorescent treponemal antibody absorption (FTA-ABS, and *T. pallidum* particle agglutination assay (TPPA), *T. pallidum* hemagglutination assay (TPHA), *T. pallidum* enzyme immunoassay (TP-EIA), chemiluminescence immunoassay (CIA), and immunoblot assay.
- *Nontreponemal specific tests* include rapid plasma reagin (RPR), venereal disease research laboratory (VDRL) and toluidine red unheated serum test (TRUST).

NICE recommendations on testing for syphilis—(1) 10-mL clotted blood sample to obtain a full syphilis screen; (2) Swab any active lesions on the genitals or elsewhere with a "flock" swab, for syphilis PCR and also for herpes simplex; (3) Screen for other STIs—chlamydia, hepatitis B/C, and human immunodeficiency virus (HIV). Definitive diagnosis of intrauterine infection is established by diagnostic testing of amniotic fluid or fetal blood, but invasive procedures are routinely not recommended due to their inherent risks.

TREATMENT

Multidisciplinary team (MDT)—genitourinary medicine physicians, neonatologists, and microbiologists. It includes antimicrobial therapy, counseling, partner notification, and safe sex advice.

World Health Organization (WHO) recommendations for treatment of syphilis in pregnancy is given in **Table 1**.

TABLE 1: WHO stagewise and trimester-wise treatment of syphilis in pregnancy.

Stage of disease	*First/second trimester*	*Third trimester*
Early disease (primary/secondary or latent <2 years)	Benzathine penicillin 2.4 MU intramuscular (IM); single dose	Benzathine penicillin 2.4 MU IM; weekly for 2 weeks/doses
Late disease (latent/unknown duration)	• Benzathine penicillin 2.4 MU IM; weekly for 3 weeks/doses • Same regimen is used in all stages of pregnancy	

If unable to tolerate intramuscular (IM) treatment, then alternative is Amoxicillin 500 mg and Probenecid 500 mg, both orally, four times per day for 14 days.

For pregnant women with penicillin allergy, desensitization may be done and treated with Penicillin, Alternatively, WHO recommends using one of the following alternative regimens:

- *Early syphilis:* Erythromycin 500 mg orally four times daily for 14 days, or Ceftriaxone 1 g intramuscularly once daily for 10–14 days, or Azithromycin 2 g once orally (when local susceptibility to Azithromycin is likely)
- *Late syphilis:* Erythromycin 500 mg orally four times daily for 30 days

During treatment, be aware of Jarisch–Herxheimer reaction, due to large numbers of *T. pallidum* being killed, which in turn releases excessive cytokines, initiating an acute inflammatory reaction. Within first 24 hours of treatment patient may have fever, rigors, and a skin rash (50% of primary syphilis, 90% of secondary syphilis, and 25% of latent disease). Treatment is IV fluids, supportive care and symptom control by Opioids, Paracetamol, and Hydrocortisone. Sometimes uterine contractions may occur, so syphilis treatment should be done under observation/admission.

Note: Diday–Kassowitz Law: If a woman with untreated syphilis has a series of pregnancies, the likelihood of infection of the fetus in later pregnancies becomes less.

Congenital syphilis may be early (first 2 years of life) or late (>2 years of birth), taken care by pediatrician. Due to ↑congenital syphilis, ACOG recommends screening all pregnant individuals serologically for syphilis at the first prenatal care visit, followed by universal rescreening during the third trimester and at birth, rather than using risk-based approach to testing.

SUGGESTED READING

1. ACOG. (2024). Screening for Syphilis in Pregnancy. [online] Available from https://www.acog.org/clinical/clinical-guidance/practice-advisory/articles/2024/04/screening-for-syphilis-in-pregnancy [Last accessed September, 2024].
2. Dewick L, Jayaprakasan K, Raouf S. Syphilis in pregnancy: identifying and managing a historic problem on the rise. Obstetr Gynaecol. 2020;22:209-16.
3. Kingston M, French P, Higgins S, McQuillan O, Sukthankar A, Stott C, et al. UK National Guidelines on the Management of syphilis 2015. Int J STD AIDS. 2016;27(6):421-46.

NOTES

NOTES

SECTION 5

Demography and Neonatal Problems

Section Authors: *Shashi Bala Arya, Parul Maheshwari, Sunaina Chandra*

CHAPTER 31

Nonimmune Hydrops (NIH)

DEFINITION

Presence of ≥2 abnormal fluid collections in fetal soft tissues and serous cavities, such as pleural effusion/pericardial effusion/ascites and skin edema, not caused by red cell alloimmunization. It is associated with severe perinatal morbidity/mortality (60%) and significant maternal risks, including maternal mirror syndrome (preeclampsia-like condition, where the mother also becomes swollen like hydropic fetus).

INCIDENCE

1 in 2,000 pregnancies, increasing due to ∵↓incidence of immune hydrops because of extensive use and availability of Anti-D for red cell isoimmunization.

ETIOLOGY

Known in ~60% cases, due to fetal, placental, and maternal pathology. Any cause of fetal cardiac or hepatic failure → ↑plasma oncotic pressure and ↑ central venous pressure (CVP) → ↑interstitial fluid and/or ↓lymphatic return associated with high capillary permeability → nonimmune hydrops fetalis (NIHF).

Main causes—fetal chromosomal/monogenic abnormalities, fetal infections (Parvovirus B19, cytomegalovirus, toxoplasmosis, and syphilis) and fetal cardiovascular problem; inborn metabolic disorders, hematological and fetomaternal hemorrhage (anemia, high output cardiac failure); extracardiac anomalies—thoracic, gastrointestinal, urogenital, lymphatic dysplasia; tumors (including chorangioma).

APPROACH

History Taking

Obstetric history—Miscarriages/fetal losses, previous NIHF or affected fetuses/infants; Family history—Consanguinity, genetic diagnoses, suspected genetic conditions, developmental delay in children/other family members, childhood, or premature adult deaths. Medical/H-recent illnesses, infectious contacts, travel, profession, risk of fetal viral infection, and likely pathogens [e.g., Parvovirus B19, cytomegalovirus (CMV), and toxoplasmosis].

History of presenting complaints—Maternal-discomfort, abdominal expansion (polyhydramnios), symptoms of preeclampsia (maternal mirror syndrome).

Clinical Examination

Blood pressure + urinalysis ± protein creatinine ratio, abdomen girth, and reflexes.

INVESTIGATIONS

Venous blood sample: Full blood count (FBC), liver function test (LFT), urea and electrolytes (U&E), coagulation, soluble Fms-like tyrosine kinase 1 (sFlt-1)/placental growth factor (PlGF) ratio or PlGF.

Imaging—2D and 3D fetal ultrasound: Middle cerebral artery peak systolic velocity (MCA-PSV), echo ± skeletal survey, fetal growth velocity, and umbilical artery pulsatility index (UAPI), placental appearance, liquor volume, ± magnetic resonance imaging (MRI). Maternal virology screen (Parvovirus B19, CMV, and toxoplasmosis immunoglobulins), hemoglobinopathy screen. Fetal investigations—Fetal deoxyribonucleic acid (DNA) obtained via chorionic villus sampling (CVS), fetal blood sampling (FBS), pleural tap, fetal hemoglobin, pleural tap, ascitic tap [fetal DNA—polymerase chain reaction (PCR) and chromosomal microarray analysis (CMA) (if normal then exome sequencing)], in second/third trimesters if MCA-PSV >1.5 multiple of the median (MoM), fetal blood sampling for anemia and transfusion, if required. In pleural effusion, fluid for virology, protein concentration and cell count (exudate/transudate), in ascites, biochemistry, and cytology [lymphoid cell counts >80% suggestive of chylous effusions, vacuolated lymphocytes sign of glycogen storage diseases, ↑ gamma-glutamyl transferase (GGT) in bowel perforation, ↓total protein in urinary ascites].

Flowchart 1: Management of first trimester NIHF.

First trimester NIHF on USG → History; index pregnancy, obstetric, family, and exposure to infections

↓

Inform about chance of miscarriage, refer to fetal medicine → USG to confirm viability and hydrops fetalis, first trimester anatomy including fetal echo, placental appearance, and feasibility of CVS

↓

Options—(1) If fetal demise/wants MTP → Counsel, arrange medical/surgical management, cytogenetics of products of conception. (2) If wants to continue pregnancy → offer diagnostic testing, MDT referral, and according to history, ultrasound, and genetic results, radiology/MRI → Involve neonatal, palliative care, neonatal/pediatric cardiologists, and clinical genetics teams—shared decision making

(CVS: chorionic villus sampling; MDT: multidisciplinary team; MRI: magnetic resonance imaging; MTP: medical termination of pregnancy; NIHF: nonimmune hydrops fetalis; USG: ultrasonography)

Flowchart 2: Management of second/third trimester NIHF.

Second/third trimester NIHF on USG → History; index pregnancy, obstetric, family, and exposure to infections

↓

Urgent assessment for fetal anemia, carry out MCA Doppler for PSV >1.5 MoM, urgent assessment in FMU → history of index pregnancy, obstetric, family and exposure to infections; detailed ultrasound for hydrops fetalis, MCA-PSV, detail anatomy including fetal echo, skeletal survey, and/or genetic sonogram, estimate fetal size and Dopplers, placental appearance

↓

If fetal anemia confirmed, counsel, provide rescue in utero transfusion, identify immune cause (maternal red-cell antibodies and susceptible fetus)

↓

Offer diagnostic testing—Amniocentesis (>15 + 0) for DNA PCR/CMA, if negative and pregnancy continuing discuss with clinical geneticist for exome sequencing (ES), infection screen, compare with booking results, PCR of amniotic fluid, if suspected fetal infection

↓

MDT referral including clinical genetics, pediatric cardiology, radiology/MRI → Involve neonatal, palliative care, neonatal/pediatric specialists and clinical genetics teams; and shared decision making if wants MTP/fetal demise—Genetic testing of cord/fetal tissue; CMA +/– ES

(CMA: chromosomal microarray analysis; DNA: deoxyribonucleic acid; ES: exome sequencing; FMU: fetal medicine unit; MCA-PSV: middle cerebral artery peak systolic velocity; MoM: multiple of the median; MRI: magnetic resonance imaging; NIHF: nonimmune hydrops fetalis; PCR: polymerase chain reaction; USG: ultrasonography)

MANAGEMENT (FLOWCHARTS 1 AND 2)

Counseling regarding poor fetal prognosis especially if <14 weeks (associated with genetic disease/CVS problems), mostly fetal demise so medical termination of pregnancy (MTP) (under section for congenital malformation) should be advised in first trimester + fetal and placental tissue for postnatal testing.

In second/third trimester, multidisciplinary team (MDT)—clinical geneticists, genomic scientists, neonatologists, and perinatal pathologists with fetal medicine unit (FMU) referral urgently to rule out anemia (MCA-PSV >1.5 MoM) and intrauterine blood transfusions if required; followed by further fetal imaging, targeted investigations, and diagnostic testing to find the cause.

Fetal therapy considered if (1) known cause of NIHF; (2) woman is committed and wants to continue the pregnancy; (3) informed consent regarding procedural risks, benefits, and alternatives; (4) a specialist MDT discussion for favorable outcome is achievable; and (5) a trained and competent fetal therapy team to perform the procedure (thoracic-amniotic shunts for pleural effusion, etc.).

Maternal therapy—if polyhydramnios—amniocentesis, indomethacin 25 mg 6-hourly till 32–34 weeks, if maternal mirror (Ballantyne) syndrome—consider delivery according to gestational age.

SUGGESTED READING

1. Khairudin D, Alfirevic Z, Mone F, Navaratnam K. Non-immune hydrops fetalis: a practical guide for obstetricians. Obstet Gynaecol. 2023;25:110-20.

CHAPTER 32

Fetal Growth Restriction

DEFINITION

Fetal growth restriction (FGR) is a multifactorial disorder due to various pathological factors resulting in failure of the fetus to thrive its growth potential. Clinically, it is defined as estimated fetal weight (EFW) and/or abdominal circumference (AC) <3rd percentile for the period of gestation irrespective of Doppler studies or between 3rd and 10th percentile with abnormal Doppler studies {abnormal uterine artery Doppler [UAD] [mean pulsatility index (PI) >95th centile]} and/or abnormal umbilical artery (UA) Doppler (absent or reversed end diastolic flow or PI >95th centile).

The FGR is broadly classified into early (<32 weeks) and late onset (≥32 weeks) based on gestational age at the time of diagnosis, in absence of congenital anomalies. Incidence—10% of all pregnancies, of these 30% are early and 70% are late onset FGR. Early FGR <32 weeks remains a challenging entity associated with an increased risk of perinatal and maternal morbidity and mortality.

Small for gestational age (SGA) are small and happy fetuses with normal fluid and Doppler studies and EFW at 3rd–10th percentile [Appropriate for Gestational Age (AGA)—fetal size between the 10th–90th centile]. (LGA—Large for Gestational Age >90th percentile).

Static growth—No forward growth velocity in EFW, or AC measured at least 14 days apart.

ETIOLOGIES

Growth restriction may occur due to maternal, placental, and fetal factors that interfere with the normal mechanisms of fetal growth. Maternal hypertension, diabetes, with vasculopathy, moderate/severe renal impairment [especially associated with hypertension], antiphospholipid syndrome (APS), systemic lupus erythematosus (SLE), anemia, smoking, alcohol, and substance abuse. Placental causes such as infarction, abruption, villitis, and mosaicism are the common ones. Cord abnormality such as increased umbilical cord coiling, length, true knot, single UA, and marginal or velamentous cord insertion. Fetal factors are chromosomal aneuploidies-aberrations and congenital malformation, certain intrauterine infections, e.g., TORCH [toxoplasmosis, others (syphilis, hepatitis B), rubella, cytomegalovirus, herpes simplex], syphilis, malaria, zika, and teratogen exposure.

RISK FACTORS

Maternal age ≥40 years, low body mass index (BMI) <18.5 kg/m^2, ethnicity (Southeast Asian, African, and Black African Caribbean), bariatric surgery, previous FGR/SGA, previous stillbirth, history of preterm birth (PTB) or second trimester loss due to placental dysfunction, previous pregnancy with placenta-mediated complications, low socioeconomic status, and poor nutrition (caffeine consumption ≥300 mg/day). Current pregnancy risks—first trimester biochemical markers—↓pregnancy-associated plasma protein A (PAPP-A)/ ↑beta-human chorionic gonadotropin (β-hCG), second trimester biomarkers— ↑ α-fetoprotein (AFP), ↑inhibin-A; mid-trimester anomaly scan—Echogenic bowel, single UA, fetal biometry EFW <10th centile; hypertensive disorders of pregnancy (HDP), antepartum hemorrhage (APH), and corona virus disease of 2019 (COVID-19) infection.

FETAL GROWTH RESTRICTION AND COMPLICATIONS

Hypoglycemia, hyperbilirubinemia, hypothermia, necrotizing enterocolitis, respiratory distress syndrome, and intraventricular hemorrhage are the neonatal morbidities associated with prematurity and FGR apart from intrauterine fetal demise, birth asphyxia, and stillbirth; Neonates at ↑ risk of neurodevelopmental disorders and metabolic syndrome.

MANAGEMENT

Treatment depends on the cause of FGR. In structurally and chromosomally normal FGR fetuses; following are the protocols to be followed: (1) Early prediction of FGR, (2) Preventive interventions, and (3) Antenatal fetal surveillance.

Early Prediction of Fetal Growth Restriction

Detailed maternal history including age, residence of high altitude, chronic hypertension, chronic kidney disease, SLE, APS, diabetic vasculopathy, and history of FGR in previous pregnancy. Low serum placental growth factor (PlGF) and PAPP-A (<5th percentile) value and high mid-trimester serum AFP [>2 multiple of the median (MoM)] and inhibin-A (>2 MoM) value done for aneuploidy can be utilized as one of the predictors for FGR in index pregnancy.

Symphysis fundal height (SFH) is recommended at each antenatal appointment >24^{+0} weeks of pregnancy (no more frequently than every 2 weeks). Fundal height measurement in cm using over the curve technique can approximate the gestational age from 16 to 38 weeks within 3 cm. The zero mark of a nonelastic tape is placed at the upper most border of pubic symphysis of a patient in a semirecumbent position with a corrected longitudinally placed uterus **(Figs. 1A and B)**. Clinical evaluation of uterine fundal height has its own limitations—uterus may be elevated in following conditions:

- Previous cesarean delivery
- Height of mother, ↑ BMI (>35 kg/m^2)
- Relative displacement of umbilicus
- Large myoma
- Multiple gestation, polyhydramnios

Correct assessment of duration of pregnancy is paramount in suspecting growth disorders. If SFH <10th centile/serial measurements demonstrate suboptimal fetal growth (no apparent fetal growth over 2 weeks) or less accurate, then refer for ultrasonography (USG) biometry and color Doppler velocimetry. Uterine artery **(Fig. 2)**: PI >95th percentile and bilateral notching detected in mid-trimester scan at 18–20 weeks' gestation (as by this time placental remodeling is completed). Those with normal UAD mid-trimester and normal fetal biometry, serial scanning for fetal biometry can commence at 32 weeks, and those with abnormal UAD can commence at 24^{+0}–28^{+6} weeks.

Preventive Interventions

Dietary modification—balanced energy/protein supplementation, stop smoking /alcohol/drugs, Aspirin 150 mg once daily at night from 12^{+0} to 36^{+6} weeks of pregnancy, 10 µg/day of vitamin D (throughout pregnancy) and 400 µg/day of Folic acid (preconception + first 3 months pregnancy) [Phosphodiesterase-5 (PDE-5) inhibitors, e.g., Sildenafil to treat FGR only in clinical trials].

Antenatal Fetal Surveillance

Most of the tests evaluate or depend on the maturity of fetal central nervous system (CNS) and its synchronicity with other systems, which would not have developed before 32 weeks. Fetal kick count done by mother is the most cost-effective modality. Nonstress test (NST), amniotic fluid index (AFI), fetal biometry, and interval growth velocity, Doppler ultrasound of the fetal arterial and venous circulation, and biophysical profile are the tests employed for fetal assessment (Gradual hypoxia theory explains us

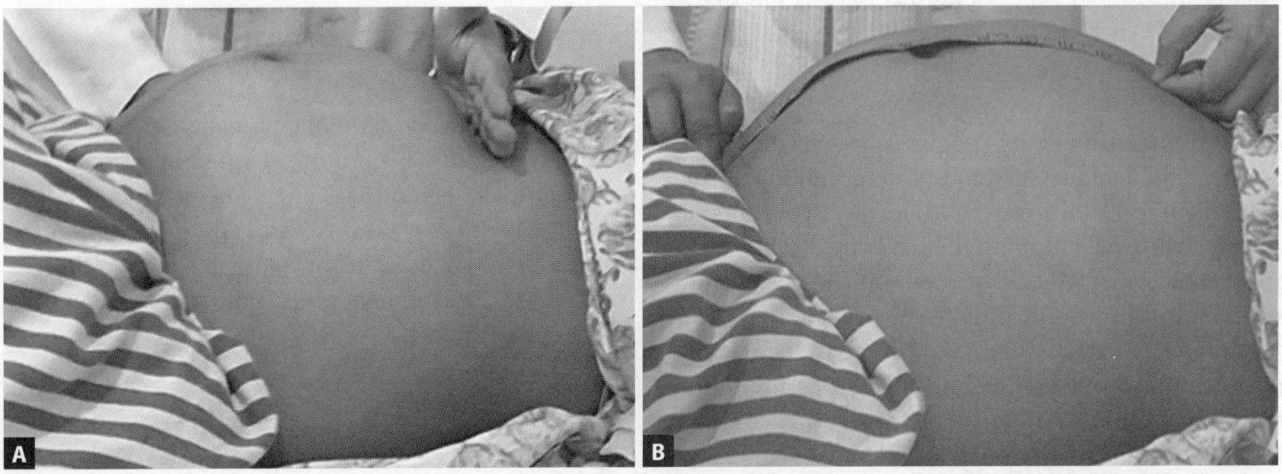

Figs. 1A and B: (A) Measuring fundal height in pregnant woman; (B) Measuring symphysio-fundal height in pregnant woman.

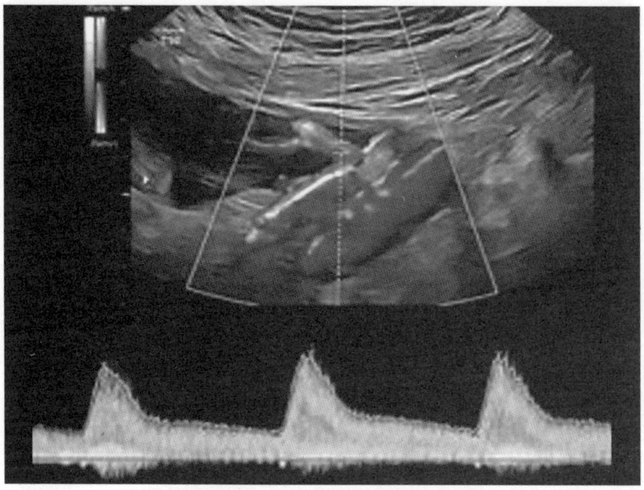

Fig. 2: Uterine artery normal wave form.

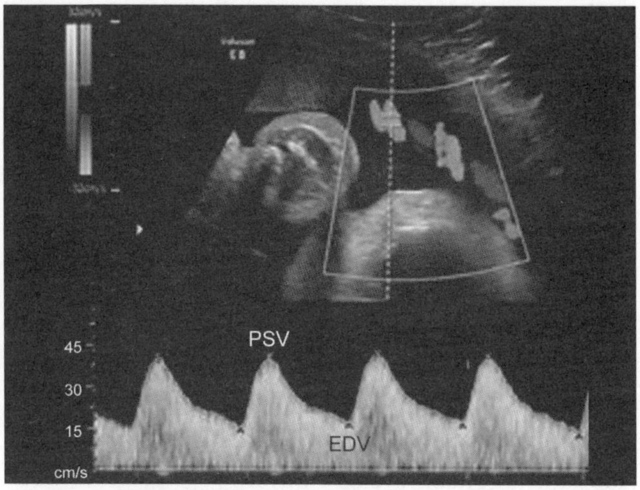

Fig. 3: Umbilical artery normal wave form. (EDV: end-diastolic velocity; PSV: peak systolic velocity)

how the biophysical activity which appear first disappear last). The art of management of FGR lies in selecting best time and mode of delivery to minimize the risk of prematurity, birth asphyxia, and stillbirth.

FOLLOW-UP OF *SUSPECTED* FETAL GROWTH RESTRICTION/SMALL FOR GESTATIONAL AGE

Book her in high-risk pregnancy clinic for antenatal care. UA PI **(Fig. 3)** and middle cerebral artery (MCA) PI **(Fig. 4)** and fetal measurements including AFI, biparietal diameter (BPD), head circumference (HC), abdominal circumference (AC), and femur length (FL) every 2 weeks till ≥37 weeks of gestation. Follow-up weekly and consider biophysical profile (BPP)/NST 1–2 times per week till 37–39 weeks of gestation. Deliver at 37–39 weeks of gestation. *Mode of delivery:* Vaginal by induction of labor (IOL).

FOLLOW-UP OF *CONFIRMED* FETAL GROWTH RESTRICTION

Increasing PI in UA reflects a progressive reduction in the placental surface area available for nutrient exchange and further deterioration as absent or reversal of flow on Doppler velocimetry. Contrary to UA, reduced fetal MCA-PI is "brain-sparing" effect in response to early fetal hypoxemia. SGA with early Doppler changes: (1) UA PI >95th percentile, (2) Cerebroplacental ratio (CPR) <5th percentile, (3) Oligohydramnios, (4) Suboptimal interval growth, and (5) Suspected preeclampsia. Advise admission, administer steroids for fetal lung maturation

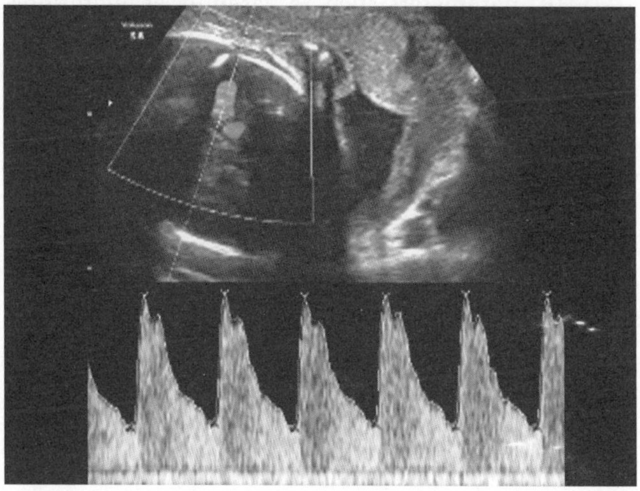

Fig. 4: Middle cerebral artery (MCA) wave form.

(between 24^{+0} and 34^{+6} weeks, ideally 48 hours before an anticipated birth), BPP/NST and Doppler [UA, MCA, and ductus venosus (DV)] twice a week, interval growth every 2 weeks; *Mode of delivery:* Cesarean section or IOL with continuous electronic fetal monitoring (CEFM) at completed 34–37 weeks by individualized approach.

FOLLOW-UP OF FETAL GROWTH RESTRICTION WITH UMBILICAL ARTERY ABSENT OR REVERSE DIASTOLIC FLOW

Risk of stillbirth is 7% with absent end-diastolic velocity (AEDF) and 19% in reversed end-diastolic velocity (REDV). It can be further minimized with strict monitoring protocol [at least twice weekly computerized cardiotocography (cCTG)/DV-a wave] with a safety net up to 0–1% in AEDV and 1–2% in REDV of UA. The median time for deterioration in AEDV is 5 days and in REDV is 2 days. Admit, administer steroids for fetal lung maturation and $MgSO_4$ for neuroprotection (offered between 24^{+0} and 29^{+6} weeks, considered up to 33^{+6} weeks), BPP/NST 1–2 times per day, Doppler (UA, MCA, and DV) every 1–2 days; *Mode of delivery:* Cesarean section.

FOLLOW-UP OF FETAL GROWTH RESTRICTION WITH ABNORMAL *DUCTUS VENOSUS* DOPPLER

Risk of stillbirth: 20%. Elevated DV pulsatility index velocity (PIV) and absent or reverse a-wave.

- Monitor with cCTG to note "short term variation" (STV) in milliseconds [cCTG evaluates fetal heart rate (FHR) parameters such as baseline, accelerations, decelerations, and variability in an objective and quantifiable way, and provides the parameter of STV in milliseconds].

If cCTG not available quantify variability in traditional way in beat-to-beat variation per minute.

Mode of delivery: Cesarean section

Postpartum: Placenta for histopathology (HPE) in FGR, counseling regarding next pregnancy prevention plans.

CONCLUSION

The FGR remains a leading contributor to perinatal mortality and morbidity in neonates. Advancements in diagnostic and therapeutic modalities has potential to improve neonatal outcome. Though no cure is available, and management is reliant on a structured antenatal surveillance program with timely intervention.

SUGGESTED READING

1. Boers KE, Bijlenga D, WJ Mol B, LeCessie S, Birnie E, G van Pampus M. Disproportionate Intrauterine Growth Intervention Trial At Term: DIGITAT. BMC Pregnancy Childbirth. 2007;7:12.
2. Cunningham F, Leveno KJ, Dashe JS, Hoffman BL, Spong CY, Casey BM (Eds). Williams Obstetrics, 26th edition. United States: McGraw Hill; 2022.
3. Growth Restriction Intervention Trial (GRIT), 2004.
4. Morris RK, Johnstone E, Lees C, Morton V, Smith G; Royal College of Obstetricians and Gynaecologists. Investigation and care of a small-for-gestational-age fetus and a growth restricted fetus (GTG No. 31). BJOG. 2024;131(9):e31-e80.
5. Symonds I, Arulkumaran S. Essentials of Obstetrics, 5th edition. London: Churchill Livingstone Publishers Pvt. Limited; 2013.
6. Truffle group (2017). The Trial of Randomized Umbilical and Fetal Flow in Europe. (TRUFFLE). [online] Available from https://truffle-study.org/. [Last accessed September, 2024].

CHAPTER 33

Neonatal Resuscitation

INTRODUCTION

In intrauterine life, fetus depends upon placenta (and cord) for respiration, which gets interrupted for 50–75 seconds at the time of uterine contraction during delivery. Majority of neonates are able to withstand this period of perinatal asphyxia, few babies may require resuscitation/support for this transition. ~10% need some intervention, 1% need extensive resuscitation. Perinatal asphyxia → progressive hypoxemia, hypercapnia, and metabolic acidosis. Clinical features depends on etiology, intensity, and duration of oxygen lack, plasma CO_2 excess and subsequent acidosis. Asphyxia livida—stage of cyanosis, asphyxia pallida—stage of shock.

Implications: Long-term neurological complications, death neonatal resuscitation (NNR): Simple, inexpensive, and cost-effective method.

For successful NNR, four factors required are:

1. *Anticipation:* Call skilled personnel
2. Adequate preparation
3. Accurate evaluation (algorithm-based)
4. Prompt initiation of support

ANTICIPATION

Risk factors:

- Maternal—age, diabetes mellitus (DM), hypertension (HTN), substance abuse, history of stillbirth/intra-uterine demise (IUD)/neonatal death (NND).
- Fetal—prematurity, postmaturity, congenital anomalies, fetal growth restriction (FGR), and multiple pregnancy.
- Antepartum complications—Placental anomalies, oligohydramnios, and polyhydramnios.
- Delivery complications—Transverse lie, breech, chorioamnionitis, meconium-stained liquor (MSL), abnormal fetal heart rate (FHR), maternal narcotics within 4 hours of birth, instrumental delivery, lower segment cesarean section (LSCS) for maternal/fetal compromise.

ADEQUATE PREPARATION

Radiant warmer is turned on and is heating. Oxygen source is open with adequate flow through the tubing. Suction apparatus tested, functioning properly. Laryngoscope is functional with bright light. Resuscitation bag and mask demonstrates an adequate seal and generation of pressure.

Suction equipment—Bulb syringe, mechanical suction and tubing, suction catheters (different sizes), feeding tube, and meconium aspirator.

Bag and mask equipment—To deliver positive pressure ventilation (90–100% O_2), face masks (term and preterm size), oxygen source with flowmeter and tubing (O_2 blender for preterm).

Intubation equipment—Laryngoscope with straight blades ("0"→preterm, "1"→term), extra bulb and batteries, endotracheal tubes and its securing device/tape, alcohol sponges, CO_2 detector, laryngeal mask airway (LMA) (transport incubator for preterm).

Medication—Epinephrine, Sodium bicarbonate, Naloxone, isotonic crystalloids— normal saline (N/S), lactated Ringer (R/L); 10% dextrose, etc., syringes with needles or puncture device for needleless system.

Miscellaneous—Gloves, personal protective equipment (PPE), radiant warmer, warm linen (1 pair) (plastic wrap for preterm), clock with seconds, firm padded resuscitation surface, stethoscope, cardiac monitor with electrodes or pulse oximeter with probe, and oropharyngeal airway.

ACCURATE EVALUATION, ALGORITHM-BASED

For uncompromised babies delayed cord clamping of at least 1 minute is recommended for placental transfusion, except when baby needs resuscitation. So, rapid clinical assessment of neonate should be done as baby is received and start the clock—Is the infant full term? Is the infant breathing or crying? Does the infant have good muscle tone? Color of baby and heart rate? → If baby is pink, active, breathing regularly, and heart rate >100: no resuscitation, routine neonatal care (keep warm, early skin-to-skin contact, and early breastfeeding).

PROMPT INITIATION OF SUPPORT

If no change, needs resuscitation → Call for help, keep the infant *warm and dry*—by changing the wet towel, to maintain the temperature 36.5–37.5°C → Assess color, tone, breathing, and heart rate and reassess every 30 seconds → clear *airway* if necessary—by placing the baby on back with head in neutral position **(Fig. 1)** to ensure straight patent airway (neither flexion nor extension—if not provide some support below shoulders so that forehead is almost parallel to the surface) and stand on head side.

Suctioning of mouth and oropharynx should be done if there is any obvious airway obstruction by mucus/blood/vernix/meconium (for tracheal obstruction—intubation and suctioning under direct visualization should be done by trained neonatologist) and stimulate → if infant is still *not breathing* give five inflation breaths using umbo-bag and mask with air (mask of appropriate size—"0" for preterm and "1" for term)—it should snugly cover nose, mouth, and chin, without any overlap of eyes, catch hold in *"C"* position—with thumb and index and *"E"* position with rest three fingers of nondominant hand, and dominant hand squeezing the bag **(Fig. 2)**.

Look for the chest rise with each squeeze, allowing the bag to reinflate fully. *Inflation* breaths are longer lasting for 3 seconds (to expel fluid out of lungs), so counting out loud helps to maintain rhythm—"1-2-3-press-1-2-3-press"—continue till five inflation breaths and reassess—color/tone/breathing and heart rate.

If there is no chest rise with first press, reassess the neck position, mask size and application—consider single person jaw-thrust/two-person airway control, consider superficial suctioning if required, connect to O_2 (5 L/min) rather than air and repeat inflation breaths → Reassess, if after 1 minute baby is still unable to breathe independently, check heart rate → if ≥60/min → ventilation breaths, if <60/min → do cardiopulmonary resuscitation (CPR), i.e., ventilation breaths + chest-compression simultaneously.

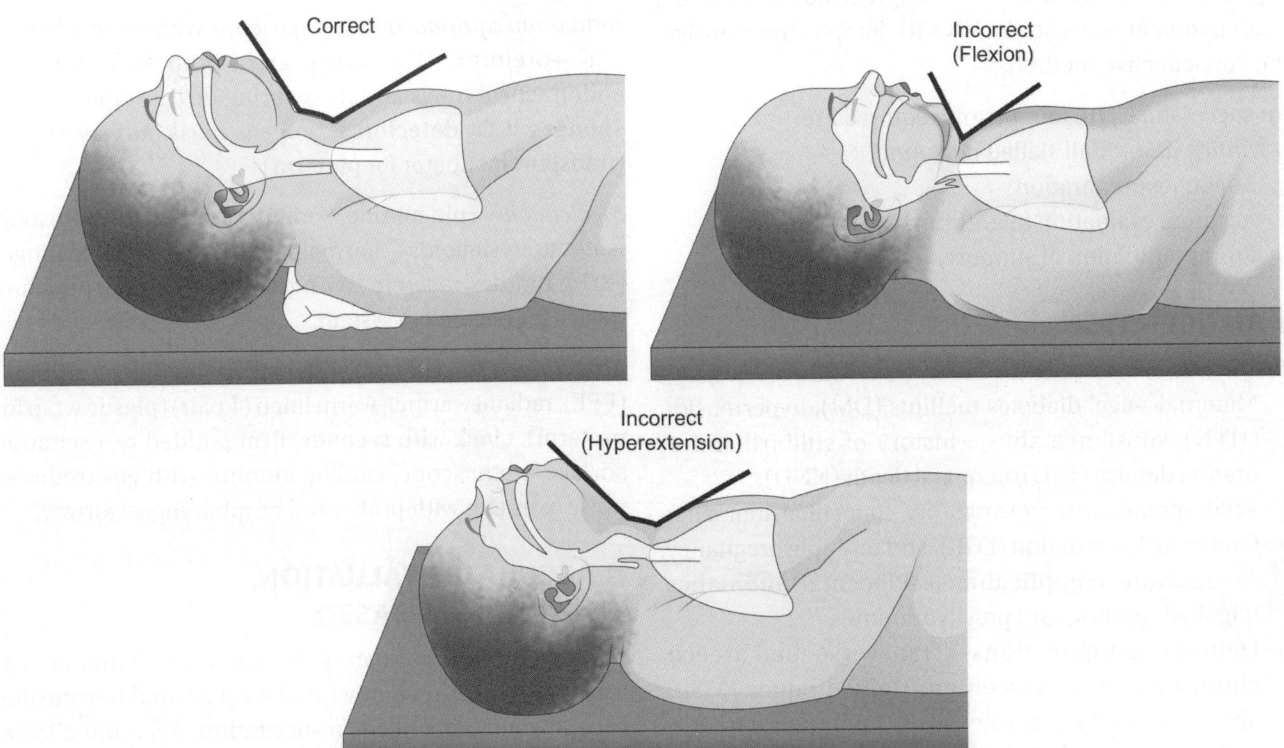

Fig. 1: Head position for neonatal resuscitation. The top panel demonstrates the correct head position with the baby positioned on the back with the neck slightly extended resulting in alignment of the posterior pharynx, larynx, and trachea, which allows unrestricted air entry.

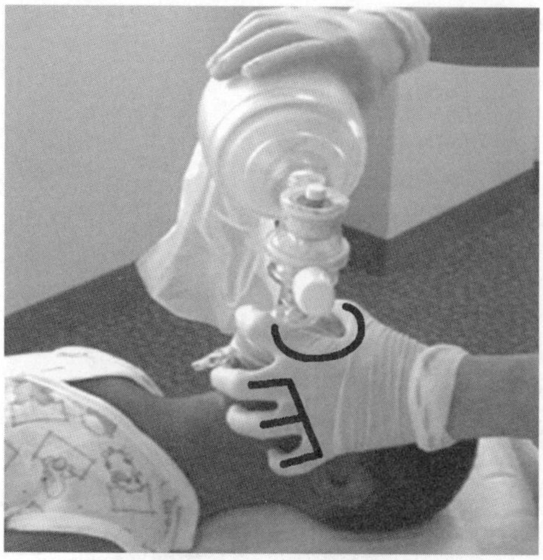

Fig. 2: Correct mask holding technique. E-C clamp technique. The hand is positioned so that the little, ring, and index fingers are spread over the mandible from the angle of the jaw forward toward the chin in the configuration of the letter "E". The jaw is then lifted, pulling the face into the mask. The thumb and forefinger are placed over the mask in the shape of the letter "C". The mask is squeezed onto the face and a seal is formed between the mask and the face.

Ventilation breaths differ from inflation in that it is short lasting for 1 second each, i.e., "1" second squeeze—"1" second release—"1" second squeeze (mimic normal pattern of breathing) → reassess after 30 seconds, stop if baby breathes independently at 30 breaths/min, if not start chest compression @ 3:1 breaths (two fingers on lower one-third of sternum below the nipple line if one person/in case of two persons → two thumbs at lower one-third of sternum with other fingers encircling the chest) **(Figs. 3 and 4)** aim to compress firmly and quickly at least one-third of depth of chest → reassess after 30 seconds → if heart rate <60, consider venous access and intravenous (IV) medication through umbilical route—Adrenaline/Sodibicarb/IV fluids along with intubation → if recovers continue postresuscitation care with close observation, if not then admit to neonatal intensive care unit (NICU). **Flowchart 1** displays the complete algorithm of NNR, which should be in every delivery room.

Golden minute—In <30 seconds: Complete initial steps—Warmth, drying, clear airway, if necessary, stimulate; next 30–60 seconds: Assess two vital characteristics—Respiration (apnea/gasping/labored/unlabored), heart rate (<100/>100 bpm).

Stop resuscitation—Newborn with no detectable heart rate, consider stopping NNR if the heart rate remains undetectable for 10–20 minutes of resuscitation, document and debrief.

NNR not indicated—Conditions with certainly early death, e.g., diaphragmatic hernia with hypoplastic lungs extreme prematurity [gestational age (GA) <23 weeks], birth weight <400 g, anencephaly, chromosomal abnormality—Trisomy 13.

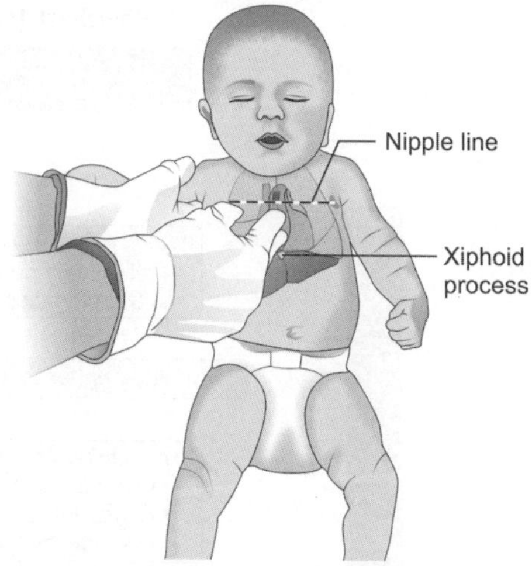

Fig. 3: Chest compression—single hand. Chest compression for infant resuscitation: Two thumb technique. Chest compressions for infants (under 1 year) may be performed with two fingers placed on the sternum just below the nipples. This picture shows the site of compressions. When the compressions are performed the two fingers used should be perpendicular to the chest and straight.

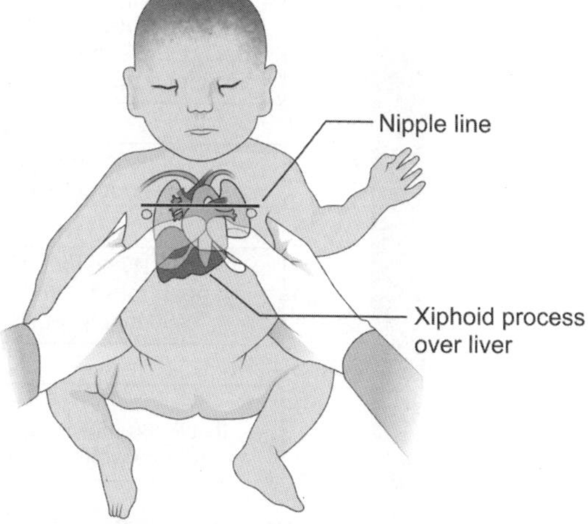

Fig. 4: Chest compression—both hands. Chest compression for infant resuscitation: Two finger technique. The thorax is encircled with the hands and cardiac compressions are performed with both thumbs. The compression site is approximately one finger's breadth below the intermammary line. The area over the xiphoid process should be avoided to prevent injury to the liver, spleen, or stomach.

Flowchart 1: Algorithm of neonatal resuscitation.

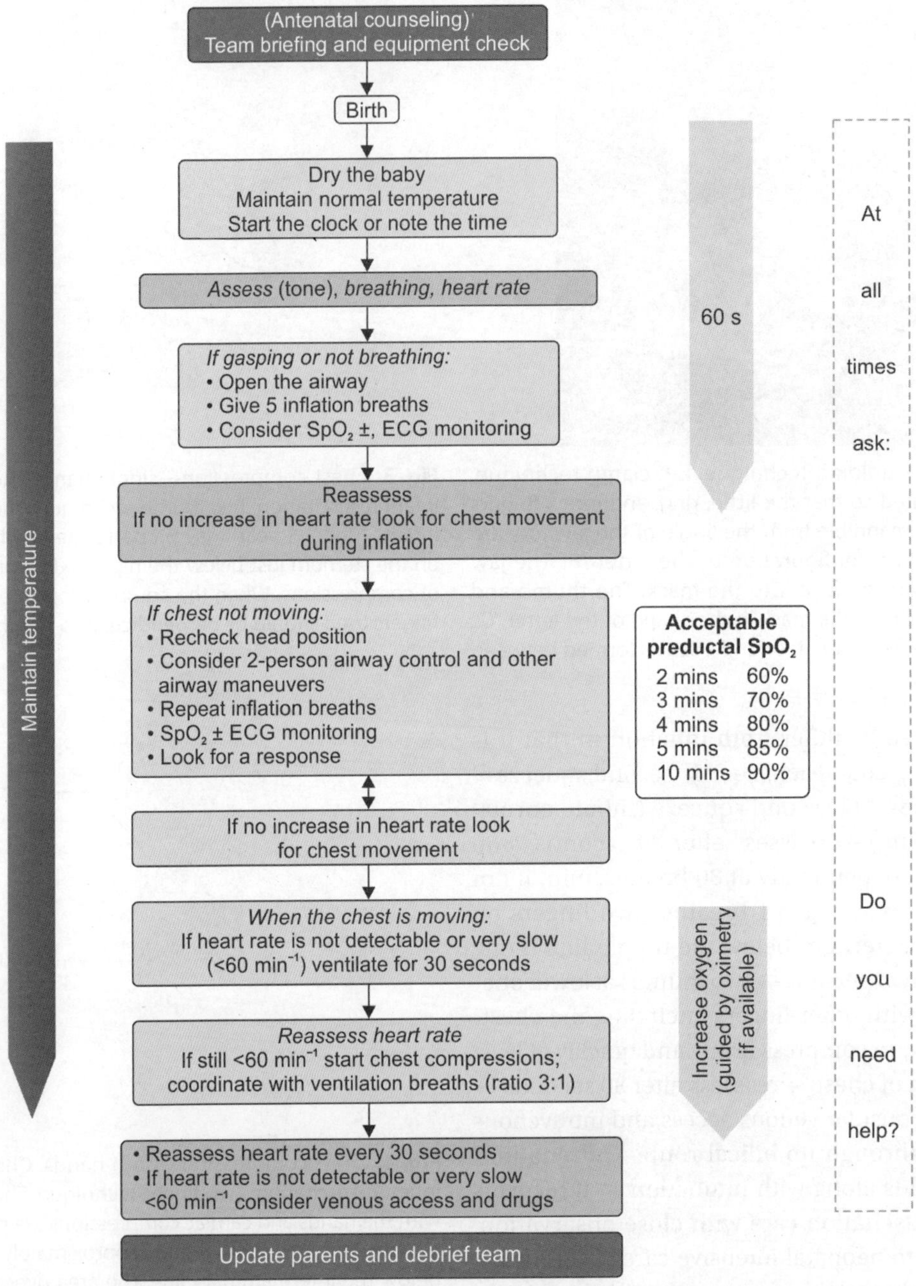

(ECG: electrocardiogram; SpO_2: oxygen saturation)

SUGGESTED READING

1. Fernandes CJ, Garcia-Prats JA, Tehrani N. Up to date Neonatal resuscitation in delivery room. [online] Available from https://medilib.ir/uptodate/show/5015 [Last accessed September, 2024].
2. Resuscitation Council, UK. 2021 Resuscitation Guidelines. [online] Available from https://www.resus.org.uk/library/2021-resuscitation-guidelines [Last accessed September, 2024].

NOTES

NOTES

SECTION 6

Menstrual Disorders

Section Authors: *Mridu Sinha, Pooja Mishra, Chanchal Choudhary*

CHAPTER 34

Premenstrual Syndrome

DEFINITION

Combination of physical (bloatedness and mastalgia) and psychological symptoms (depression, anxiety, irritability, loss of confidence, and mood swings) that cause significant impairment of daily functioning of an individual during the luteal phase of the menstrual cycle, and abate as menstruation begins, followed by a symptom-free week.

INCIDENCE

40% (5–8% severe)

TYPES

- Core premenstrual disorders (PMD)
- "Variant" PMDs are of four subtypes: (i) Premenstrual exacerbation of an underlying disorder, (ii) Non-ovulatory PMDs, (iii) Progestogen-induced PMDs, and (iv) PMDs with absent menstruation.

ETIOLOGY

Two theories include the following:

1. Some are "sensitive" to progesterone and progestogens as serum concentrations of estrogen/progesterone are same in those with or without premenstrual syndrome (PMS).
2. Implicates the neurotransmitters serotonin and γ-aminobutyric acid (GABA) as serotonin receptors are responsive to estrogen and progesterone, and selective serotonin reuptake inhibitors (SSRIs) are proven to reduce PMS symptoms; GABA levels are modulated by metabolite of progesterone, allopregnanolone, and in PMS allopregnanolone levels appear to be reduced.

DIAGNOSIS

Prospective symptom diary [daily record of severity of problems (DRSP)] for two consecutive menstrual cycles, if inconclusive then gonadotropin-releasing hormone (GnRH) analogs used for 3 months to confirm it, that inhibits ovulatory cycles and causes a complete hormonal suppressive effect.

MANAGEMENT

Multidisciplinary team (MDT)—general practitioner, a general gynecologist or a gynecologist with a special interest in PMS, a mental health professional—psychiatrist, clinical psychologist or counselor, and a dietician.

- Patient education about premenstrual symptoms and self-help coping strategies.
- *Complementary therapies*—for *physical symptoms*—*routine exercise*, reflexology, *acupuncture, Vitex* agnus castus, *Ginko* biloba, saffron, vitamin B6, *Ca (1,000–1,200 mg/day)*/vitamin D, and evening Primrose oil have shown some benefits in certain trials but their dose/strength and safety not established, and they may interact with conventional medicines. Cognitive behavioral therapy (CBT) may also help for *affective* PMS.
- Nonsteroidal anti-inflammatory drugs (NSAIDs) for premenstrual pain symptoms.
- *Nonhormonal medical management:* SSRIs (Escitalopram, Citalopram), either luteal (favored more) or continuous dosing, should be first-line pharmaceutical management in *affective* PMS. Most common, dose-dependent side-effects—nausea, asthenia, somnolence, fatigue, decreased libido, and sweating. Also, if given on a continuous basis, should be discontinued gradually to avoid withdrawal symptoms.
- Diuretics like Spironolactone can be used in women with PMS to treat physical symptoms.
- Hormonal medications like Drospirenone-containing combined oral contraceptive (COC), if given continuously for 3 months is more effective than cyclical therapy. Alternative is percutaneous estradiol combined with cyclical progestogens [along with effective contraception—barrier/intrauterine contraceptive device (IUCD)]. With estradiol, insufficient data on long-term effects on breast and endometrial tissue.

- For prevention of endometrial hyperplasia, with percutaneous Estradiol, a cyclical 10–12-day course of oral/vaginal progesterone or long-term progestogen with the Levonorgestrel-releasing intrauterine system (LNG-IUS) 52 mg should be used. Lowest possible dose of progesterone/progestogen is recommended to minimize progestogenic adverse effects. Micronized progesterone is less likely to reintroduce PMS-like symptoms and should be considered as first-line.
- Low dose Danazol (200 mg BD) is effective in the luteal phase for breast symptoms, but as it has potential irreversible virilizing effects, contraception should be advised during treatment due to its potential virilizing effects on female fetuses.
- GnRH analogs should be reserved for most *severe, refractory* PMS and not recommended routinely unless used to establish and/or support a diagnosis or treat particularly severe cases, especially before surgical treatment to predict the response. If >6 months, add-back hormone therapy, with continuous combined hormone replacement therapy (HRT) (or Tibolone) is recommended; bone mineral density (BMD) by dual-energy X-ray absorptiometry (DEXA) every year, and stopped if bone density declines significantly.
- Progesterone/progestogens/LNG-IUS alone not recommended.
- Surgical treatment—hysterectomy and bilateral oophorectomy should be considered when medical management failed, long-term GnRH analogue treatment is required or other gynecological conditions indicate surgery. But surgery should not be done without preoperative use of GnRH analogs as a test of cure and to ensure that HRT is tolerated especially if <45 years of age and done for PMS alone.
- No role of endometrial ablation and hysterectomy with conservation of the ovaries. Also, bilateral oophorectomy alone (without removal of the uterus) will necessitate the use of progestogen as part of subsequent HRT regimen and this will ↑ risk of PMS-like symptoms (progestogen-induced PMD).
- **First line:** Exercise, CBT, vitamin B_6, combined new generation pill (cyclically or continuously), continuous or luteal phase (day 15–28) low dose SSRIs, e.g., Citalopram/Escitalopram 10 mg.
- **Second line:** Estradiol patches (100 µg) + micronized progesterone [100 mg or 200 mg (day 17–28), orally or vaginally] or LNG-IUS 52 mg, high dose SSRIs continuously or luteal phase, e.g., Citalopram/Escitalopram 20–40 mg.
- **Third line:** GnRH analogs + add-back HRT (continuous combined estrogen + progesterone (e.g., 50–100 µg estradiol patches or 2–4 doses of estradiol gel combined with micronized progesterone 100 mg/day) or Tibolone 2.5 mg.
- **Fourth line:** Surgical treatment ± HRT.

SUGGESTED READING

1. Green LJ, O'Brien PMS, Panay N, Craig M, on behalf of the Royal College of Obstetricians and Gynaecologists. Management of premenstrual syndrome. BJOG. 2017;124: e73-e105.
2. Management of Premenstrual Disorders ACOG Clinical Practice Guideline No. 7. Obstet Gynecol. 2023;142(6): 1516-33.

CHAPTER 35

Heavy Menstrual Bleeding

DEFINITION

Excessive menstrual blood loss that interferes with woman's physical, emotional, social, or material quality of life, unrelated to pregnancy and occurs only during reproductive years.

ABNORMAL UTERINE BLEEDING (ACUTE OR CHRONIC)

Defined as bleeding from uterine corpus that is abnormal in regularity, volume, frequency, or duration and occurs in absence of pregnancy. Acute abnormal uterine bleeding (AUB) refers to an episode of heavy bleeding that requires immediate intervention to prevent further blood loss. Acute AUB may occur spontaneously or within the context of chronic AUB (abnormal uterine bleeding present for most of the last 6 months).

CAUSES AND ETIOLOGY

Table 1 displays the International Federation of Gynecology and Obstetrics (FIGO) classification of AUB.

DIAGNOSIS: HISTORY

- *Menstrual history*—including current bleeding episodes, intermenstrual bleeding, any other symptoms—pelvic pain and/or pressure symptoms, that might suggest uterine cavity abnormality, histological abnormality, adenomyosis, or fibroids.
- *Past medical history*—systemic illness, current/recent medication, coagulation disorders, hemophilia, and platelet function disorders, leukemia, liver failure, and medications, such as anticoagulants or chemotherapeutic agents, that can impair coagulation.
- *Family history*—in particular coagulopathy, hormone sensitive cancers.
- *Social history*
- Rule out any iatrogenic cause of bleeding, any previous treatment for heavy menstrual bleeding (HMB).

TABLE 1: PALM-COEIN classification.

PALM: Structural causes	*COEIN: Nonstructural causes*
Polyp	Coagulopathy
Adenomyosis	Ovulatory dysfunction
Leiomyoma	Endometrial
Malignancy and hyperplasia	Iatrogenic
	Not yet classified

INVESTIGATIONS

All women of reproductive age group should have a urine pregnancy test (UPT).

Laboratory Tests

- *Full blood count*—anemia (loss ≥120 mL menstrual blood), sepsis, and leukemia.
- *Blood grouping and cross-matching (±UPT) in acute blood loss.*
- *Thyroid function test, liver function test (LFT), serum iron, total iron-binding capacity (TIBC) if symptomatic specifically.*
- *Testing for bleeding [Von Willebrand factor (vWf), clotting factor VIII test (f.VIII)]/coagulation disorder [prothrombin time (PT)/activated partial thromboplastin time (APTT)/international normalized ratio (INR)/serum fibrinogen]*—if history of HMB since menarche or personal/family history of coagulation disorder.
- *Imaging, histology, and microbiology:*
    - *Ultrasound pelvis* for assessing endometrium and adnexa.
    - *Cervical smear*
    - *High vaginal and endocervical swabs* for infection (*Chlamydia trachomatis*)
    - *Pipelle endometrial biopsy*—in persistent intermenstrual bleeding, >45 years old, evidence of unopposed estrogen exposure [obesity, polycystic ovary syndrome (PCOS)], and/or failure of pharmacological treatment.

TABLE 2: First-line medication.

Drug	*Dose*	*Duration*	*Efficacy*	*Side-effects*
NSAIDs	500 mg TDS	For 3 days	About 25–50% reduction in menstrual blood loss	GI discomfort, diarrhea, nausea, vomiting, headache, and dizziness
Tranexamic acid	1 g TDS or QDS	To be taken for up to 4 days; maximum 4 g per day	50% reduction in menstrual blood loss	Diarrhea (reduce dose if occurs), nausea, and vomiting

(GI: gastrointestinal; NSAIDs: nonsteroidal anti-inflammatory drugs)

- *Hysteroscopy:* When ultrasound identifies pathology or if their history suggests submucosal fibroids, polyps, or endometrial pathology due to symptoms of persistent intermenstrual bleeding or risk factors for endometrial pathology. It should be "see-and-treat" hysteroscopy in a single setting.
- *Endometrial biopsy* at time of hysteroscopy who are at high risk of endometrial pathology, e.g., persistent intermenstrual or persistent irregular bleeding or infrequent heavy bleeding who are obese or have PCOS, on Tamoxifen, or in whom treatment for HMB is unsuccessful.

MANAGEMENT

Acute AUB—prompt initial assessment for signs of hypovolemia and hemodynamic instability → intravenous (IV) access with a single or two large bore IV lines, and preparation for blood transfusion and clotting factor replacements → evaluate for most likely etiology of acute AUB.

Definitive treatment given after discussing risks and benefits of different options, impact on her fertility whether wants to retain her uterus. Aim of management is to improve a woman's quality of life.

- *Nonpharmacological:* Regular exercise and maintenance of a healthy body mass index (BMI) should be recommended to every adolescent. A high BMI will increase the risk of ovulatory dysfunction and subsequent heavy or irregular menstrual loss. A healthy diet will also help limit iron deficiency anemia, raise energy levels, and improve quality of life.
- *Pharmacological:*
  - *Nonhormonal options* **(Table 2)** for HMB management.
  - *Hormonal options:*
    - In acute bleeding, IV conjugated equine estrogen usually tried first.
    - Combined hormonal contraceptives (CHC)—multidoses may be required.
    - Levonorgestrel-releasing intrauterine system (LNG-IUS)—first-line as more effective than oral medication in treatment for HMB, also works as contraceptive. A 90% reduction in menstrual blood loss seen over 12 months use. It is effective for 5 years. Wait for at least six cycles to see the benefits of treatment.
    - Cyclical oral progestogens
    - *Ulipristal acetate:* LFT should be measured before giving this drug.

Contraindications for hormonal treatment—breast cancer (current/past), active/past DVT/pulmonary embolism, deranged LFT, smoking, uncontrolled hypertension (HTN), diabetes mellitus (DM) with vasculopathy, migraine with aura, cerebrovascular disease, ischemic heart disease, and major surgery with prolonged immobilization.

SURGICAL TREATMENT

- *Endometrial ablation:* It is suitable for women who no longer wish to conceive (although they will need to continue using contraception), and possibility of premalignant and malignant endometrial lesions are ruled out. It can reduce HMB by up to 80%.
- *Uterine artery embolization*—done in females who have preferably completed child bearing but are unfit for surgery (morbid obesity, DM, and multiple medical problems) or not willing to undergo surgery.
- *Hysterectomy:* It can be subtotal or total hysterectomy, done either by open or laparoscopic routes. It should be considered when other treatment options have failed or the woman no longer wishes to retain her uterus and fertility.
- *Myomectomy:* Done in cases of fibroid causing infertility in reproductive age groups. It can be open

myomectomy, laparoscopic assisted myomectomy, and robot assisted.

SUGGESTED READING

1. ACOG committee opinion no. 557: Management of acute abnormal uterine bleeding in nonpregnant reproductive-aged women. Obstet Gynecol. 2013;121(4): 891-6.
2. NICE guideline [NG88]. (2018). Heavy menstrual bleeding: assessment and management. [online] Available from https://www.nice.org.uk/guidance/ng88 [Last accessed September, 2024].

CHAPTER 36

Fibroid (Leiomyoma)

DEFINITION

Myoma/leiomyoma/fibromyoma, most common benign monoclonal tumors that originate from the smooth muscle cells of uterus. *Incidence:* 30–40%.

TYPES (FIG. 1)

- *Submucosal* [International Federation of Gynecology and Obstetrics *(FIGO)—0, 1, 2*]: Located just beneath the endometrial lining.
- *Intramural (FIGO—3, 4, 5):* Within the uterine wall.
- *Subserosal (FIGO—6, 7):* On the outer surface of the uterus.
- *Cervical (FIGO—8):* Located in the cervix.
- *Pedunculated:* Attached to the uterus by a stem-like structure.

RISK FACTORS

- Age—most common between 35 and 45 years.
- Parity (>20 weeks)—Nulliparous or low parity (↑parity, ↓chances ∵ repeated involution postdelivery)
- Race/ethnicity—Black race (↑X2-3 fold) (? early menarche)
- Menstrual cycle—Early menarche
- Genetic predisposition—Family history
- BMI ↑—Obesity
- Medical disorders—Diabetes, hypertension (HTN)
- Chronic psychological stress/major life events

↓*Risk* associated with ↑parity, ↑physical activity, ↑intake of dietary vitamin A/green vegetables, (?) Depot Medroxyprogesterone Acetate (DMPA)/Levonorgestrel-releasing intrauterine system (LNG-IUS), and cigarette smoking (inhibition of aromatase).

PATHOPHYSIOLOGY

Exact cause unknown, but factors believed to play role are:

- *Genetic mutations:* Changes in multiple genes that differ from those in typical uterine muscle cells.
- *Hormonal influences:* Estrogen and progesterone promote fibroid growth by binding to receptors in the fibroid tissue.

Leiomyoma subclassification system

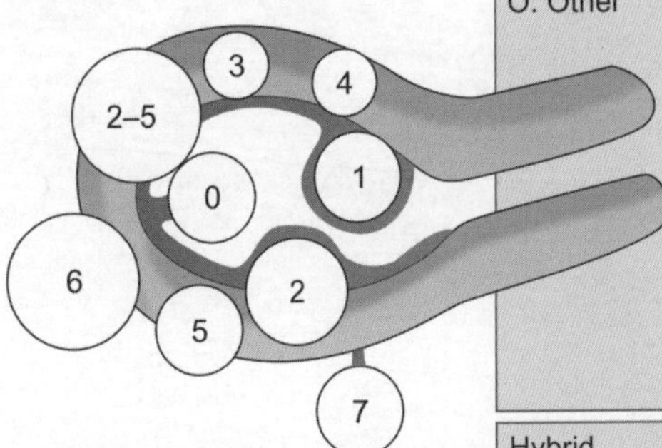

SM: Submucosal	0	Pedunculated intracavitary
	1	<50% intramural
	2	≥50% intramural
O: Other	3	Contacts endometrium; 100% intramural
	4	Intramural
	5	Subserosal ≥50% intramural
	6	Subserosal <50% intramural
	7	Subserosal pedunculated
	8	Other (specify, e.g., cervical, parasitic)
Hybrid leiomyomas (impact both endometrium and serosa)	2–5	Two numbers are listed separated by a hyphen. By convention, the first refers to the relationship with the endometrium while the second refers to the relationship to the serosa. One example is below Submucosal and subserosal, each with less than half the diameter in the endometrial and peritoneal cavities, respectively

Fig. 1: FIGO classification of fibroids. (FIGO: International Federation of Gynecology and Obstetrics)

- *Extracellular matrix (ECM):* Increased ECM in fibroids makes them fibrous.

Role of Estrogen in Development of Fibroid

Rarely found before puberty, commonly in reproductive age and regresses after menopause; Higher incidence in nulliparous/low parity women as compared to multiparity in which due to repeated process of involution in puerperium get absorbed; obese women due to ↑aromatase enzymes leading to ↑peripheral conversion of androgens to estrogens by aromatization; ↑during pregnancy—↑concentrations of estrogen receptors in leiomyoma than myometrium, common in fourth decade due to anovulatory cycles associated with high or unopposed estrogen.

Fibroid Pathology

- *Grossly*—Multiple, distinct, globular, pinkish white, firm capsulated masses protruding from surrounding myometrium, pseudo capsule—compressed adjacent myometrium.
- *Microscopy*—Nonstriated smooth muscle fibers arranged in interwoven bundles of varying size in whorl-like pattern, intermixed with connective tissue in between.

Pathological Variants

- Intravenous leiomyomatosis
- Leiomyomatosis peritonealis dissemination (LPD)
- Secondary changes—Hyaline, fatty, calcific, necrosis, or red degeneration in pregnancy.
- Leiomyosarcoma—~0.5%, common in fifth decade, with atypical mitotic figures.

CLINICAL PRESENTATION

- *Commonly asymptomatic*—incidentally diagnosed on imaging
- *Abnormal uterine bleeding*—30–50%, heavy/prolonged menstrual bleeding [common with submucous fibroids (SMF)] due to ↑surface area; impaired endometrial hemostasis or molecular dysregulation of angiogenic factors leading to ↑vascularity, thinning and ulceration of overlying endometrium, endometrial hyperplasia, altered uterine contractility—inhibits usual ability of uterus to contract during menses.
- *Anemia* due to excessive blood loss.
- *Pelvic pain*—backache; torsion, infection, expulsion, red degeneration, and vascular complication.
- Dysmenorrhea—Spasmodic as well as congestive.
- Bulk-related pressure symptoms—pelvic pressure/pain, urinary tract or bowel obstruction, or venous compression.
- Lump in abdomen
- Urinary symptoms—urgency, frequency, difficulty in emptying bladder, and rarely complete urinary obstruction.
- Bowel symptoms—constipation, intermittent intestinal obstruction.
- Rapid growth—pregnancy and malignancy.
- Prolapsed fibroid through cervix—mass, bleeding, ulceration, and infection.
- Infertility—2–10% cases—due to irregular cavity interfering with sperm transport, endometrial changes interfering with implantation.
- Endocrine effects—polycythemia [erythropoietin (EPO)], hypercalcemia [parathyroid hormone (PTH)—related protein], hyperprolactinemia.

EXAMINATION

- Assess the severity, duration, and impact on quality of life.
- G/E—Anemia (MC-iron deficiency) due to prolonged heavy bleeding, rarely fever in degeneration.
- P/A—If >12 weeks size, irregular (according to number/site, and size), firm, nodular, nontender, arising from pelvis, lower limit cannot be reached, mobile from side-to-side, dull on percussion.
- P/S—Cervix may be pulled higher up/submucosal prolapsing fibroid.
- P/V—Uterus enlarged, nodular, firm and irregular according to number, site, and size of fibroid; Differential diagnosis from ovarian tumor → Uterus not felt separately from fibroid, cervical movement transmitted to tumor, no groove sign/notch felt between tumor and uterus.
- P/R—May help in difficult cases.

CONFIRMATION OF DIAGNOSIS

- *Transvaginal ultrasound (TVS):* First-line investigation—hypoechoic well-circumscribed round lesions, peripheral calcification with distal shadowing.
- Saline infusion sonography—Help differentiate submucous from intramural fibroids.

- *Hysteroscopy:* Uterine cavity and protruding intramural/SMF.
- *Magnetic resonance imaging (MRI):* Most effective imaging modality for diagnosis of fibroid, precise fibroid mapping, and characterization. Also:
  - Differential diagnosis from adenomyosis/adenomyoma/leiomyosarcoma
  - Differential diagnosis from adnexal pathology
  - Done before *uterine artery embolization (UAE)*
- *Hysterosalpingogram (HSG):* Done for infertility evaluation. Coincidental finding of filling defects.
- *Contrast enhanced ultrasound*—as an alternative to MRI, limited evidence.
- Lab tests—Full blood count (FBC) for anemia, urine pregnancy test (UPT), endometrial sampling to rule out coexistent premalignant/malignant endometrial lesions.

D/Dx—Pregnancy, adenomyosis, endometrial polyp, ovarian tumor, endometriosis, tubo-ovarian mass.

INDICATIONS OF EXPECTANT MANAGEMENT

- Asymptomatic incidental fibroids (spontaneous shrinkage)
- Attempting pregnancy
- Size <12 weeks and stable for 1 year
- Approaching menopause (loss of hormonal support)
- During pregnancy (postpartum remodeling)
- *Prerequisites:* Compliant patients
  - Regular periodic evaluation for any new symptoms every 6–12 months
  - History taking and routine P/S and P/V examination for evidence of fibroid growth
  - Baseline imaging with TVS/MRI to compare regression/progression

MEDICAL MANAGEMENT

- Not definitive treatment, only for symptom controls/build-up of hemoglobin (Hb)
- For symptomatic relief from pain—nonsteroidal anti-inflammatory drugs (NSAIDs), Paracetamol (PCM)
- Decrease menstrual blood loss—Tranexamic acid, Ethamsylate
- Iron, Folic acid, vitamin C, protein for treatment of anemia
- Preoperatively to decrease the size of fibroid
- Drugs used:
  - Combined oral contraceptive pill (COCP) or progestogens [oral/intrauterine contraceptive device (IUCD)]
  - Antiprogesterone (Mifepristone)
  - Gonadotropin-releasing hormone (GnRH) analogs (agonists—Leuprolide; antagonists—Elagolix, Relugolix, and Linzagolix) with or without add-back therapy.
- Selective estrogen receptor modulators (SERMs) (Ormeloxifene) and selective progesterone receptor modulator (SPRM) (Ulipristal).

Patients not desiring fertility [for heavy menstrual bleeding (HMB)]—medical treatment → first line—COCP/LNG-IUS (if cavity not disturbed)/high dose oral progestogen; → second line—GnRH agonists/antagonists/mifepristone/ulipristal/UAE/hysteroscopic resection if submucosal fibroid; → third line MRI guided focused ultrasound surgery (MRgFUS)/high intensity focused ultrasound (HIFU)/endometrial ablation/myomectomy/hysterectomy.

Patients desiring fertility—Myomectomy (laparoscopic/open) or for SMF—hysteroscopic resection with preoperative counseling of risks and benefits.

SURGICAL MANAGEMENT

- *Hysterectomy → abdominal/vaginal/laparoscopic-assisted vaginal hysterectomy (LAVH), total laparoscopic hysterectomy (TLH)*
- *Myomectomy → abdominal/vaginal/hysteroscopic/laparoscopic*

Newer Modalities

- Laparoscopic myolysis
- Uterine artery embolization
- MRI guided focused ultrasound surgery
- High intensity focused ultrasound

SUGGESTED READING

1. Williams textbook of Gynecology, 4th edition.

CHAPTER 37

Menopause and Hormonal Replacement Therapy

DEFINITION

Menopause (MP) is permanent cessation of menstruation at the end of reproductive life due to loss of ovarian follicular activity. Retrospective definition of 12 months of no periods. Age range of 45–55 years, average 50 years. Premature menopause <40 years, early MP 40–45 years, late/delayed MP if menstruation continues beyond 55 years.

Menopausal transition (climacteric/perimenopause)—transitional phase of 3–4 years before and up to 1 year after last menstruation, during which genital and other organs involute in response to cessation of gonadal activity, caused by fluctuating hormone levels [↓Estrogen and Progesterone, ↑ follicle-stimulating hormone (FSH)].

RISK FACTORS

Genetic family history, malnutrition, chemoradiation (alkylating agents), smoking and alcohol, ovarian/uterine (hysterectomy) surgery, drugs—Gonadotropin-releasing hormone (GnRH), Heparin, Corticosteroids, Clomiphene (anti-OGN) when given over prolonged period (>6 months) can cause estrogen deficiency. → early MP. No relation → age of menarche, last pregnancy, number of pregnancy, lactation, OCP, race, height, weight, and socio-economic status

MENOPAUSAL SYMPTOMS

Menstrual symptoms, vasomotor symptoms, osteoporosis, cardiovascular disease, cerebrovascular disease, psychological changes, urogenital atrophy, skin and hair changes, sexual dysfunction, dementia and cognitive decline (vasomotor and vaginal symptoms are cardinal symptoms of MP).

MENSTRUAL SYMPTOMS

Three classic ways in which the menstrual period ceases are:

1. Sudden cessation
2. Gradual diminution in the amount of blood loss with each regular period until menstruation stops.
3. Gradual increase in spacing of periods until they cease for at least a period of 1 year. If irregular with/without excessive bleeding, malignancy should be ruled out.

VASOMOTOR SYMPTOMS

"Hot flushes"—sudden feeling of extreme heat especially on upper body, face, and neck, followed by profuse sweating, most severe at night and during times of stress, lasts few seconds to several minutes (1–5). It varies in frequency and duration and in majority it lasts for 1–2 years, 25% may experience for >5 years. Other signs and symptoms—headache, palpitation, fatigue, anxiety, weakness, sleep disturbances, irritability, lack of concentration [↑systolic blood pressure (SBP), basal metabolic rate (BMR)], skin temperature rise—finger and toes (10–15°C), perspiration, flushing and chills due to cutaneous vasodilation.

ETIOLOGY

Thermoregulatory center associated with GnRH center. Normally, fluctuations of core body temperature within thermoneutral zone (0.4°C), does not trigger compensatory autonomic mechanisms but during menopausal transition this thermoregulatory zone is narrowed and becomes more sensitive to subtle changes in core body temperature due to ↑ central noradrenergic activation. Reduction in estrogen → ↓ inhibitory presynaptic α_2 adrenergic receptors, ↑ hypothalamic norepinephrine and serotonin release → lowers set point in thermoregulatory nucleus and allow heat loss mechanisms to be triggered by subtle changes in core body temperature.

Genitourinary Changes

Normally, OGN maintains epithelium of vagina, urethra, and urinary bladder which becomes atrophy, ↓ sensitivity of urethral smooth muscle and ↓ periurethral collagen due to OGN deficiency. Signs and symptoms are dryness, dysuria, frequency, urge/stress incontinence, recurrent urinary tract infection (UTI), dyspareunia, atrophic vaginitis, infections, bleeding, pruritus, leucorrhea. Loss of tone of pelvic floor muscles causes pelvic relaxation and u-v descent.

Skin and hair changes—Estrogen deficiency → rapid loss of collagen, loss of elasticity, causes wrinkling—"Purse string" around mouth and "Crow feet" around eyes. Loss of pubic and axillary hair.

DIAGNOSIS

According to the National Institute for Health and Care Excellence (NICE)—in a healthy woman >45 years with menopausal symptoms, diagnose **perimenopause** if **vasomotor symptoms with irregular periods**, and menopause if no periods at least for 12 consecutive months (not on any hormonal contraception), *without* any FSH levels [no role of anti-Müllerian hormone (AMH)/inhibin/Estradiol/antral follicle count (AFC), and ovarian volume]. Use FSH to diagnose MP if between 40 and 45 years with menopausal symptoms and irregular periods, or <40 years to rule out premature ovarian insufficiency (POI).

MANAGEMENT

Prevention—Spontaneous menopause—unavoidable, artificial MP due to surgery or radiation should be delayed/prevented.

Counseling regarding physiologic events and reassurance. Avoidance of possible triggers such as spicy foods, caffeine, smoking, and alcohol may help.

Lifestyle modifications such as exercise (aerobic, sustained, regular exercise such as swimming or running, or low-intensity exercise, such as yoga), lighter clothing, sleeping in a cooler room, cool drinks, and reducing stress may help to manage hot flushes.

Complementary therapies—Phytoestrogens are non-steroidal compounds that are synthesized by plants, protect against ultraviolet light and are involved in the transport of nutrients across the stem, such as isoflavones and lignans. Soya, flaxseeds, and red clover are the richest sources of phytoestrogens. Herbal remedies—black cohosh, ginseng, *Genko* biloba, St John's wort, etc., but their safety, efficacy, and purity is unknown, and they can interact with medicines for conditions such as breast cancer, epilepsy, heart disease, or asthma.

Alternative therapies such as acupressure, acupuncture, reflexology, or homeopathy; complementary therapy such as aromatherapy; "bioidentical" hormones, local vaginal lubricants and moisturizers, may help some but more research required regarding its safety.

Nonhormonal medical treatment—Clonidine, Gabapentin, selective serotonin-reuptake inhibitors (SSRI)-Paroxetine, Thiazide, serotonin and norepinephrine reuptake inhibitors (SNRI)—Venlafaxine. Common side-effects—dry mouth, insomnia/somnolence, drowsiness, nervousness, constipation, sweating, etc.

Psychological treatment—Cognitive behavioral therapy (CBT) for low mood or anxiety related to MP.

HORMONAL REPLACEMENT THERAPY

Indications—Relief of menopausal symptoms, prevention of osteoporosis, and maintain quality of life. Special groups are premature ovarian insufficiency (POI), gonadal dysgenesis, surgical, or radiation menopause. Currently, the primary reason to prescribe hormonal replacement therapy (HRT) in postmenopausal women is for the relief of symptoms associated with estrogen deficiency.

Benefits of HRT—Improvement of vasomotor symptoms (70–80%), and urogenital atrophy, ↑ bone mineral density (BMD), ↓risk of vertebral and hip fracture, ↓colorectal cancer and possibly cardio-protection.

Risks of HRT—Endometrial cancer, breast cancer, venous thromboembolism (VTE), coronary heart disease (CHD), stroke, adverse effect on lipid metabolism, and dementia.

Contraindications of HRT—Undiagnosed genital tract bleeding, OGN-dependent tumors, history of VTE, active liver disease, and gallbladder disease.

Assessment Prior to Starting Hormonal Replacement Therapy

- Assess menopausal state and symptoms—stage of MP (peri-, postmenopausal), time of the last menstrual period, current (or history of) bleeding patter, presence/absence of acute menopausal symptoms.
- *Current contraception*—Continue contraception for 1 year after the last menstrual period in women over 50 years old, or for 2 years in women under 50 years old.
- *Check for contraindications*—Hormone-dependent malignancy, active or recent arterial thromboembolic

disease, venous thromboembolic disease, and whether the woman is on long term anticoagulation, current pregnancy, severe active liver or renal disease, un-investigated abnormal vaginal bleeding, and acute intermittent porphyria.

- Family history/personal history—Cardiovascular disease/osteoporosis/venous thromboembolism/ breast cancer, bowel cancer, and ovarian cancer.
- *Check risk factors for coronary heart disease:* Hypertension, diabetes mellitus, family history of premature myocardial infarction or stroke, cigarette smoking, sedentary lifestyle, and obesity
- Check risk factors for osteoporosis—Medical history, history of fragility fracture, and maternal history of osteoporosis, and/or fragility fractures.
- What does the woman want? Does she want to take HRT? If not, what alternatives would she prefer?
- Discuss healthy lifestyle options to prevent osteoporosis and cardiovascular disease.

Monitoring during HRT—GE, pelvic examination, blood pressure (BP), breast examination + mammography, cervical cytology, transvaginal sonography (TVS)-endometrial thickness (ET) (<5 mm), hysteroscopy/dilation and curettage (D&C) in irregular bleeding, serum estradiol <100 pg/mL.

Preparations available—Lowest effective dose, short period of time (5 years)—Conjugated OGN—0.625–1.25 mg + Medroxyprogesterone Acetate (MPA)—2.5–5 mg/day; OGN alone—hysterectomized, cyclic OGN and added PGN (second half) or continuous OGN + PGN, subdermal implants, gel, patch, cream, Levonorgestrel-releasing intrauterine system (LNG-IUS); Tibolone (**Table 1 and Flowchart 1**). Recently, a combined daily oral preparation

TABLE 1: Commonly used hormonal replacement therapy (HRT) types.

Sequential combined cyclical HRT	Estrogen daily plus progesterone/ progestogen for 10–14 days every 28–30 days cycle	Short exposure to progesterone/progestogen cyclical withdrawal bleeding
Sequential long cycle HRT	Estrogen daily for 12 weeks plus progesterone/progestogen added in the last 14 days	Higher dose less frequent exposure to progesterone/ progestogen withdrawal bleeding every 3 months
Continuous combined HRT	Estrogen plus progesterone/progestogen administered together continuously	Continuous exposure to progesterone/progestogen no withdrawal bleeding
Continuous progestogen regimen: Tibolone	Synthetic steroid with estrogenic, androgenic, and progestational activity	Continuous exposure to progestational effects no withdrawal bleeding

Flowchart 1: Selection of hormonal replacement therapy (HRT).

The selection of hormonal regimens for symptomatic women and outline of follow-up

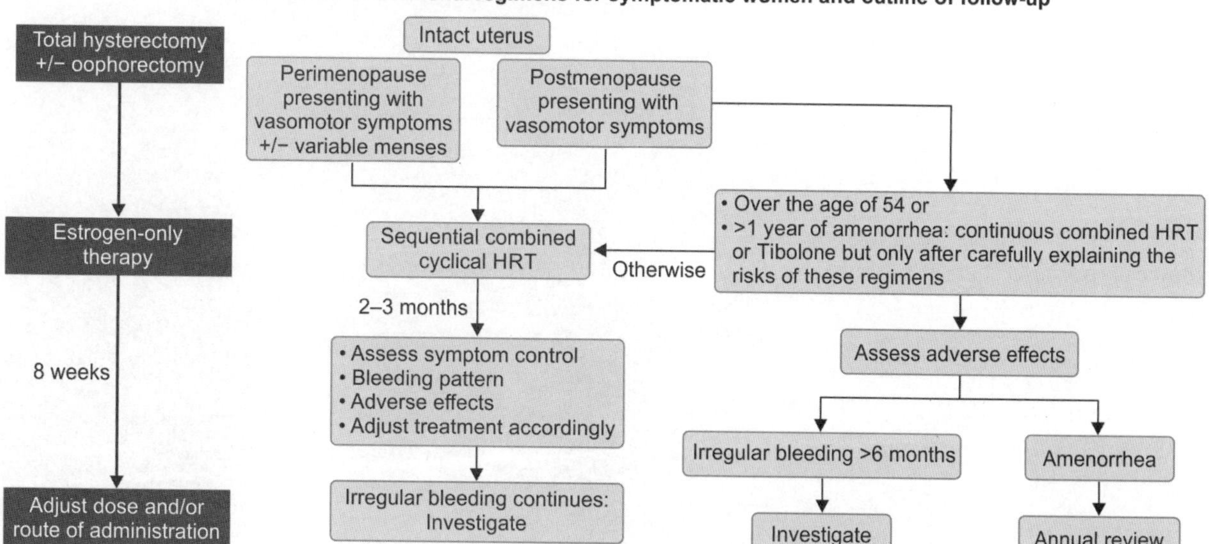

of conjugated estrogen and Bazedoxifene has been approved by the food and drug administration (FDA) for vasomotor symptoms, and to prevent osteoporosis in postmenopausal women with a uterus. FDA approved Ospemifene, a novel estrogen agonist and estrogen antagonist for vaginal atrophy without stimulating the endometrium for moderate-to-severe dyspareunia.

If combined HRT started before MP or within 12 months of last period then a "cyclical" combined HRT should be offered giving regular monthly withdrawal bleeds. If combined HRT started >12 months after last period, then woman is offered "continuous" combined HRT (bleed-free HRT). If patient had a hysterectomy then estrogen-only HRT will be offered.

Women who notice a low sex drive after the MP may be offered Testosterone, linked to sex drive in both men and women.

Follow-up—At 3 months, then yearly if no adverse effects, some may have slight irregular bleeding during first 3 months, but if persists >3 months then it should be investigated. Common side-effects are—breast tenderness, vaginal bleeding, bloating, and headaches.

SUGGESTED READING

1. ACOG Practice Bulletin PB Number 141: Management of menopausal symptoms. Obstet Gynecol. 2014;123(1): 202-16.
2. NICE guideline [NG23]. (2015). Menopause: diagnosis and management. [online] Available from https://www.nice.org.uk/guidance/ng23 [Last accessed September, 2024].
3. RCOG. (2018). Treatment for symptoms of the menopause. [online] Available from https://www.rcog.org.uk/en/patients/menopause/ [Last accessed September, 2024].

NOTES

NOTES

SECTION 7

Infertility and Endocrinology

Section Authors: *Ruchica Goel, Mridu Sinha, Sunaina Chandra*

CHAPTER 38

Premature Ovarian Insufficiency

(*Synonyms:* Premature menopause/premature ovarian failure/primary ovarian insufficiency).

DEFINITION

Clinical syndrome characterized by menstrual disturbances (oligomenorrhea/amenorrhea) due to loss of ovarian activity <40 years of age.

PREVALENCE

1%, ethnicity/family history. Modifiable risk factors are—gynae surgical practice [total abdominal hysterectomy with bilateral salpingo-oophorectomy (TAH + BSO)], lifestyle—smoking, treatment for malignant and chronic diseases.

DIAGNOSIS

The European Society of Human Reproduction and Embryology (ESHRE) Guideline Development Group (GDG) recommends the following diagnostic criteria:

- Oligo/amenorrhea for at least 4 months
- A ↑ follicle-stimulating hormone (FSH) level >25 IU/L on two occasions >4 weeks apart.

CAUSES

- Chromosomal and genetic defects—X chromosome (structural/aneuploidy), e.g., Turner syndrome (pure < mosaic), fragile-X premutation, presence of Y chromosome.
- Autosomal gene mutations—galactosemia, blepharophimosis epicanthus ptosis syndrome (BPES).
- Autoimmune ovarian damage—Addison's disease, autoimmune polyendocrine syndrome (APS), celiac disease, inflammatory bowel disease (IBD), thyroid diseases, hypoparathyroidism, type 1 diabetes mellitus (DM), and nonendocrine autoimmune diseases, systemic lupus erythematosus (SLE), Sjogren's syndrome, Rheumatoid arthritis (RA), immune thrombocytopenia (ITP), autoimmune hemolytic anemia (AIHA), and pernicious anemia.
- Infection—mumps, human immunodeficiency virus (HIV), herpes zoster, cytomegalovirus, tuberculosis, malaria, varicella, and shigella.
- Iatrogenic—radiotherapy, chemotherapy (alkylating agents), surgery [TAH + BSO, bilateral (B/L) endometriomas]
- Environmental—smoking, alcohol, and malnutrition.
- Idiopathic

CLINICAL FEATURES

May be asymptomatic, primary/secondary amenorrhea, abnormal uterine bleeding (AUB) or may present with symptoms typical of the menopause, such as hot flushes and night sweats (estrogen deficiency), vaginal symptoms—dyspareunia and dryness, altered urinary frequency, low libido, lack of energy, sleep disturbance, mood changes, poor concentration, stiffness, and dry eyes.

DIAGNOSTIC WORKUP

Karyotyping, fragile-X, test for Y chromosome material, autosomal genetic tests, antibodies—adrenocortical antibodies (ACA)/21-hydroxylase antibodies (21-OH Ab), thyroid peroxidase antibodies (TPO-Ab) + thyroid function test (TFT), serum prolactin; pelvic ultrasonography.

IMPLICATIONS

Associated with ↓ life expectancy, due to cardiovascular disease, so advised no smoking, take regular exercise, and maintain a healthy weight. 5% chance of spontaneous pregnancy, so contraception advised to avoid pregnancy. And those who want pregnancy—in vitro fertilization (IVF) with oocyte donation is an option. If pregnant, high-risk pregnancy (HRP) due to obstetric [small-for-gestational-age (SGA)/pregnancy-induced hypertension (PIH)/postpartum hemorrhage (PPH)] and nonobstetric complications, so multidisciplinary team (MDT) [e.g., cardiologist (Turners), medicine, and endocrinologist] involved. ∵↓body mass index (BMI), ↑risk of fracture, referral to orthopedician for further treatment (bisphosphonates, etc.) and monitoring bone mineral density (BMD) by DEXA scan. In Turner syndrome—Cardiovascular (CVS) risk factors should be assessed at diagnosis and annually monitored [blood pressure (BP), no smoking, weight, lipid profile, fasting plasma glucose, and HbA1c].

MANAGEMENT

Psychological and emotional counseling because of impaired self-esteem and emotional distress—cognitive behavioral therapy (CBT) and patient and family education.

Lifestyle modification, i.e., healthy lifestyle—weight-bearing exercise, avoidance of smoking, maintain normal body weight by a balanced diet with calcium (Ca) and vitamin D, hormone replacement therapy (HRT) and local vaginal estrogens (effective in genitourinary symptoms).

MDT—endocrinologist (for thyroid, adrenal disease), genetic medicine, cardiologist, orthopedician, neurologist, and menopause specialist.

Hormone replacement therapy with 17β-estradiol (preferred to ethinyl estradiol or conjugated equine estrogens) + micronized progesterone (or MPA/LNG-IUS) is ideal, and has strongest evidence of endometrial protection for oral cyclical combined treatment. It should be continued till normal age of menopause, i.e., 50–51 years with annual monitoring. This not only treats symptoms of estrogen deficiency but also have a role in primary prevention of diseases of the cardiovascular system and for bone protection.

Local estrogens may be given in addition to systemic HRT. Lubricants are useful for treatment of vaginal discomfort and dyspareunia for those not using HRT or contraindicated.

Hormone replacement therapy has not been found to increase the risk of breast cancer before the age of natural menopause. It also can be given to women with BRCA1/2 mutations but without personal history of breast cancer after prophylactic BSO.

For endometriosis, which required oophorectomy, combined estrogen/progestogen therapy is effective for treatment of vasomotor symptoms and may reduce the risk of disease reactivation.

Hormone replacement therapy contraindicated in breast cancer survivors.

Transdermal treatment for migraine, severe hypertension (HTN), history of venous thromboembolism (VTE)/thrombophilias, and obese/overweight.

If *androgen* (Testosterone for loss of libido) therapy is commenced, treatment effect should be evaluated after 3–6 months and should possibly be limited to 24 months.

Pregnancy options—Referral to a reproductive endocrinology and infertility specialist. IVF with oocyte donation, embryo donation, and adoption (no role of ovulation induction).

SUGGESTED READING

1. ACOG Committee Opinion CO Number 605. (2014). Primary Ovarian Insufficiency in Adolescents and Young Women. [online] Available from https://www.acog.org/clinical/clinical-guidance/committee-opinion/articles/2014/07/primary-ovarian-insufficiency-in-adolescents-and-young-women [Last accessed September, 2024].
2. ESHRE. (2015). Guideline on Management of women with premature ovarian insufficiency. [online] Available from https://www.eshre.eu/Guidelines-and-Legal/Guidelines/Management-of-premature-ovarian-insufficiency.aspx [Last accessed September, 2024].

CHAPTER 39

Male Infertility

DEFINITION OF INFERTILITY

Failure to conceive with in ≥1 years (6 months if female age >35 years) of regular unprotected intercourse during fertile period. Incidence—15%, i.e., 1:7 couples.

Two types include:

1. *Primary:* Have never conceived (1:8 couples).
2. *Secondary:* Had been pregnant once but thereafter cannot conceive with in one or more years of regular unprotected intercourse during fertile period (1:6 couples).

Causative factors—Male factor only in 10–20%, combined male and female factors 30–40%.

CAUSES

Age: Decreases >35 years and more pronounced >50 years (∴ semen donors' age kept <40 years).

Environmental, occupational, and lifestyle factors—obesity, exposure to heat, X-rays, heavy metals (lead, mercury), glycol ethers (highly volatile compounds used as solvents) and pesticides; exposure to electromagnetic waves emitted from mobile phones (dose-dependent); sedentary lifestyle, heavy alcohol, tobacco smoking, cannabis, cocaine, Amphetamines, and opiates consumption.

PRETESTICULAR (<1%)

- *Hypothalamic disease:* Gonadotrophin deficiency (Kallman syndrome), genetic syndromes of reduced gonadotropin-releasing hormone (GnRH) secretion (Prader-Willi syndrome, Laurence-Moon-Biedl syndrome).
- *Pituitary disease:* Pituitary insufficiency (tumors like craniopharyngioma, or its treatment like radiation, surgery, and head trauma), hyperprolactinemia, exogenous hormones (anabolic steroids, glucocorticoid excess, and hyper- or hypothyroidism), and hemochromatosis.

TESTICULAR

- Congenital, genetic, chromosomal (Klinefelter syndrome 47, XXY), Y chromosome microdeletions, Noonan syndrome (male Turner syndrome 45, XO), other, bilateral cryptorchidism.
- Acquired, injury (orchitis, torsion, and trauma), varicocele, systemic disease (renal failure, liver failure), chemotherapy, radiotherapy, testicular tumors, Idiopathic.

POST-TESTICULAR

- Congenital, cystic fibrosis, congenital absence of the vas deferens (CAVD), Young's syndrome.
- Acquired, vasectomy, infection (chlamydia, gonorrhea), iatrogenic vasal injury.
- Disorders of sperm function or motility, immotile cilia syndrome, maturation defects, immunological infertility, Globozoospermia.
- Sexual dysfunction, timing and frequency, erectile/ejaculatory dysfunction, Diabetes mellitus, multiple sclerosis, and spinal cord/pelvic injuries.

APPROACH

History Taking

- *Fertility history:* Previous pregnancies—with current and previous partners, duration of infertility, and previous infertility treatments.
- *Sexual history:* Puberty onset, sexual development history, loss of body hair/↓shaving frequency, erection or ejaculation problems, frequency of intercourse, and loss of libido.
- *Genetic disorders:* Cystic fibrosis, Klinefelter syndrome.
- *Medical history:* Recent pyrexia/chronic illness, systemic illness—diabetes mellitus, cancer, infection, history of major head trauma/surgery/radiation, infection [mumps/sinopulmonary, sexually transmitted infections (STI)]

- *Surgical history:* Undescended testes, orchidopexy, hernia repair, testicular trauma, torsion, pelvic, bladder, or retroperitoneal surgery.
- *Medication:* Nitrofurantoin, Cimetidine, Sulfasalazine, Spironolactone, α-blockers, Methotrexate, Colchicine, Amiodarone, Antidepressants, Phenothiazines, and chemotherapy.
- *Social history:* Alcohol, smoking, anabolic steroids, recreational drugs, exposure to ionizing radiation, chronic heat exposure, aniline dyes, pesticides, and lead exposure.

PHYSICAL EXAMINATION

Height, weight, body mass index (BMI), blood pressure, any signs of ↓ body hair or gynecomastia [symptoms of androgen deficiency], thyroid dysfunction, or Cushing syndrome; Urologist referral for—testicular size (mean volume <15–20 mL with orchidometer/length <3.6 cm in longest axis) and consistency, if impalpable, the groin should be examined; presence and normality of the vasa differentia, epididymis should be examined for distension or induration, engorgement of the pampiniform plexus of veins in the scrotum is indicative of a varicocele (feeling of a "bag of worms" with a Valsalva maneuver), penile (micropenis, hypospadias), and prostatic abnormalities or seminal vesicle enlargement by per rectum (PR) examination.

INVESTIGATIONS

Semen analysis: The National Institute for Health and Care Excellence (NICE) recommends semen analysis according to the World Health Organization (WHO) **(Table 1)**. If an abnormality is detected a repeat semen analysis should be done >3 months, or sooner (>3 days) if the initial test shows azoospermia. Clear instructions regarding the period of abstinence, method of production and transport of specimen to the laboratory should be provided and the sample should be analyzed within an hour of collection because sperm motility decreases after ejaculation.

Low ejaculate volumes <1.5 mL may indicate retrograde ejaculation, obstruction, androgen deficiency, incomplete collection, or anejaculation. No evidence for antisperm antibodies/seminal fructose level/postcoital testing of cervical mucus.

Endocrine tests: Follicle-stimulating hormone (FSH), luteinizing hormone (LH), testosterone (between 8 and 10 AM) and prolactin should be measured in men with sperm counts of <5 million/mL. ↓Testosterone levels with ↑FSH and LH indicate primary testicular failure whereas ↓Testosterone levels in combination with ↓LH and FSH levels indicate a central defect with secondary hypogonadism. Azoospermia in combination with normal hormone levels suggests an obstruction.

TABLE 1: World Health Organization (WHO) Semen parameters 5th percentile reference limit—comparison.

Semen parameters	*WHO-2010 (5th edition)*	*WHO-2021 (6th edition)*
Semen volume	>1.5 mL	>1.4 mL
Semen concentration × 10^6/mL	≥15 million	≥16 million
Total sperm no × 10^6/ejaculate	≥39 million	≥39 million
Total motility%	≥40%	≥42%
Progressive motility%	≥32%	≥30%
Nonprogressive motility%	1%	1%
Immotile%	22%	20%
Vitality%	≥58%	≥54%
Normal forms%	≥4%	≥4%
Leukocytes	1 × 10^6/mL	1–2 × 10^6/mL

Genetic evaluation: In severe oligospermia (<5 million/mL) or azoospermia, Klinefelter syndrome (47, XXY), microdeletion on long arm of the Y chromosome (Yq), that includes the azoospermia factor (AZF) locus, with three subregions: AZFa, AZFb, and AZFc (good prognosis for surgical sperm recovery), cystic fibrosis gene [associated with congenital bilateral absence of the vas deferens (CBAVD)].

Imaging: Transrectal ultrasonography (USG) for obstructive azoospermia, scrotal ultrasound in testicular tumor, with Doppler in varicocele may help.

Testicular biopsy in severe oligospermia and azoospermia, also facilitates sperm recovery for intracytoplasmic sperm injection (ICSI).

Sperm function test: Sperm penetration assay (SPA), hemizona assay (HZA), sperm deoxyribonucleic acid (DNA) fragmentation, sperm chromatin structure assay (SCSA), sperm chromatin dispersion (SCD) test, TUNEL (terminal deoxynucleotidyl transferase-mediated dUTP nick end-labeling) assay and single cell gel electrophoresis (COMET) assay, to assess sperm DNA integrity.

MANAGEMENT

Lifestyle Management

↑Physical activity and weight loss for obesity, diet with ↑vegetables, fruits, fish, poultry, cereals and low-fat dairy and ↓processed meat, full-fat dairy products, alcohol, coffee, and sugar-sweetened beverages. Vitamins and antioxidants may help, whereas smoking cessation, decrease if heavy/chronic alcohol/coffee consumption, stress management by cognitive behavioral therapy, psychotherapy, and fertility counseling and support. There is an association between elevated scrotal temperature and reduced semen quality, but it is uncertain whether wearing loose-fitting underwear improves fertility.

Treatment of endocrine and systemic disorders, ± gonadotropin replacement therapy, e.g., prolactinoma even after its appropriate treatment for 6–12 months is not responding then gonadotropin may be added. Any causative drugs should be stopped, treatment of ejaculatory failure can restore fertility.

Defect in spermatogenesis—if with low testosterone and high LH/FSH symptoms of testicular failure then assisted reproductive techniques (ART) is considered, if with normal hormonal levels then obstructive causes should be evaluated. No effective therapy for severe oligospermia/ azoospermia, can be offered ART with surgical retrieval [testicular sperm aspiration (TESA)/percutaneous epididymal sperm aspiration (PESA)/testicular sperm extraction (TESE)] with in vito fertilization (IVF)/ICSI or donor IUI. Surgical repair of varicocele only for symptomatic grade-3, conflicting evidence for minor degree/antibiotics for leukospermia/Clomiphene/ aromatase inhibitors/rhFSH in idiopathic male infertility. Genetic counseling and testing should be offered prior to ICSI and ART, as ART is the only potential effective treatment for most causes of male infertility.

SUGGESTED READING

1. Karavolos S, Panagiotopoulou N, Alahwany H, Martins da Silva S. An update on the management of male infertility. Obstet Gynaecol. 2020;22:267-74.
2. Karavolos S, Stewart J, Evbuomwan I, McEleny K, Aird I. Assessment of the infertile male. Obstet Gynaecol. 2013; 15:1-9.
3. NICE Clinical guideline [CG156]. Fertility problems: assessment and treatment. [online] Available from https://www.nice.org.uk/guidance/cg156 [Last accessed September, 2024].

CHAPTER 40

Ovarian Hyperstimulation Syndrome

DEFINITION

Ovarian hyperstimulation syndrome (OHSS) is a potentially serious iatrogenic complication of fertility treatment, in which pharmacological ovarian stimulation is done to increase the number of oocytes and thereby embryos during assisted reproductive technology (ART). It is associated with significant physical and psychosocial morbidity, and may lead to death in severe cases.

INCIDENCE

Mild—One-third of in vitro fertilization (IVF) cycles, combined moderate and severe 3–8%.

ETIOLOGY

Exposure of hyperstimulated ovaries [controlled ovarian hyperstimulation (COH) by follicle-stimulating hormone (FSH)] to human chorionic gonadotropin (hCG)/luteinizing hormone (LH) leads to the production of proinflammatory mediators, like vascular endothelial growth factor (VEGF) which causes ↑vascular permeability and prothrombotic effect. This leads to loss of fluid from intravascular to the third space, manifesting as ascites or, pleural and pericardial effusions; in severe cases resulting in hypovolemia [with ↓serum osmolality and decreased sodium—paradoxical combination due to "reset" of the osmotic thresholds of vasopressin and thirst to lower osmolality and sodium levels], with loss of 20% blood volume.

RISK FACTORS

Preexisting → young age, polycystic ovary syndrome (PCOS), previous ovarian hyperstimulation syndrome (OHSS), basal AMH >3.3 ng/mL, AFC >8. Related to ovarian response → multiple (>20) intermediate follicles >10 mm, high/rapidly ↑serum estradiol >3,500 pg/mL, ↑ number oocytes retrieved, hCG given for trigger/luteal phase, pregnancy.

Prevention: Gonadotropin-releasing hormone (GnRH) antagonist protocol with GnRH agonist trigger, coasting, cycle cancellation, freeze all embryos, i.e., cryopreservation [frozen embryo transfer (FET)], Progesterone (PGN) for luteal phase support, adjuvants such as Metformin, dopamine agonists—Cabergoline.

CLINICAL FEATURES

"Early" OHSS presents within 7 days of the hCG injection associated with an excessive ovarian response, "late" OHSS presents ≥10 days after the hCG injection, due to endogenous hCG from an early pregnancy (more severe). Symptoms are nonspecific and no diagnostic tests, hence differential diagnosis from other causes—ovarian torsion or cyst rupture, pelvic infection, pelvic abscess, appendicitis, bowel perforation, and ectopic pregnancy.

History—time of onset of symptoms relative to trigger, medication used for trigger (hCG or GnRH agonist), number of follicles on final monitoring scan, number of eggs collected, were embryos replaced and how many, and polycystic ovary syndrome.

C/O—abdominal bloating, abdominal discomfort/pain, need for analgesia, nausea, and vomiting, breathlessness, inability to lie flat, or talk in full sentences, ↓urine output, leg swelling, vulval swelling, associated with thrombosis.

O/E-G/E: Dehydration, edema (pedal, vulval, and sacral); pulse, blood pressure (BP), respiratory rate (RR), body weight, Chest—pleural effusion, pneumonia, pulmonary edema.

P/A: Ascites, palpable mass, and peritonism; abdomen girth.

INVESTIGATIONS

Full blood count (FBC), hematocrit (Hct) (hemoconcentration), C-reactive protein (CRP) (severity), urea and electrolytes (↓Na ↑K), ↓serum osmolality (hypo-osmolality), liver function test (LFT) (↑enzymes,

↓albumin), coagulation profile (↑fibrinogen, ↓antithrombin), hCG (to determine outcome of treatment cycle) if appropriate. *Ultrasonography (USG):* Ovarian size, pelvic and abdomen free fluid, and ovarian Doppler to rule out torsion. Severe cases—arterial blood gas (ABG), D-dimers, echocardiogram (ECG), chest X-ray (CXR), computed tomography pulmonary angiography (CTPA), or ventilation-perfusion (V/Q) scan.

Classification of severity of OHSS: Being dynamic condition, level of severity may change.

Mild OHSS "ovarian hyper-responders": Abdominal bloating/distension, mild abdominal discomfort/pain, mild nausea/vomiting/diarrhea, bilateral ovarian size usually <8 cm (no biochemical abnormality).

Moderate/severe/critical OHSS can be "self-limited" or "with significant comorbidities."

Moderate OHSS: Moderate abdominal pain/discomfort, nausea ± vomiting, USG suggestive of ascites, ovarian size usually 8–12 cm; ↑Hct >41%, ↑white blood cell (WBC) >15,000/mL, ↓proteins.

Severe OHSS: Clinical ascites (± hydrothorax), severe pain abdomen, intractable nausea/vomiting, rapid weight gain >1 kg in 24 hours, pleural effusion, dyspnea, oliguria (<300 mL/day or <30 mL/h), Hct >45%, Na+ <135 mmol/L, osmolality <282 mOsm/kg, K+ >5 mmol/L, serum albumin <35 g/L, and ovarian size usually >12 cm.

Critical OHSS: Tense ascites/large hydrothorax, Hct >55%, WBC >25,000/mL, oliguria/anuria (renal failure), thromboembolism, acute respiratory distress syndrome (ARDS), arrhythmia, pericardial effusion, massive hydrothorax, sepsis, and disseminated intravascular coagulation (DIC).

MANAGEMENT

In most cases OHSS is self-limiting and requires supportive management and monitoring while awaiting resolution. Outpatient department (OPD) for mild-to-moderate cases and inpatient department (IPD) ± intensive care unit (ICU) for severe and critical cases. Verbal and written information should be provided to patient.

OPD: Avoid heavy physical activity, daily—input/output charting, weight and AG charting; drink to thirst at least 1–2 liters a day, Paracetamol/Codeine for analgesia (NSAIDs, diuretics, contraindicated), dopamine agonists—Cabergoline (0.5 mg/day), culdocentesis/paracentesis for symptomatic relief from ascites. Monitoring every 2–3 days but if **worsening** features—↑abdominal distension and pain, shortness of breath, ↑heart rate (HR) or ↓blood pressure (BP), ↓urine output (<1 liter/24 hours) or positive fluid balance (>1 liter/24 hours), ↑weight (>1 kg/day) and AG, Hct >45%, urgent review, hospitalization, antiembolism stockings, or low-molecular-weight Heparin (LMWH).

IPD: Multidisciplinary team (MDT), admit severe cases (ICU for critical), close monitoring by modified early warning score (MEWS) [to guide admission to high dependency unit (HDU)], daily—weight and AG, intake-output (I/O) charting, blood investigations—CBC, blood urea nitrogen (BUN), creatinine, electrolytes, LFT, CRP, transvaginal ultrasound (TVUS) (as needed for ovarian size and ascites), CXR, ECG, and central venous pressure (CVP).

Supportive care, intravenous (IV) hydration—isotonic crystalloid solution—normal saline (NS)/Ringer's lactate (RL) [IV Hydroxyethyl Starch (HES)/25% albumin if no improvement in Hct/UO with crystalloids], culdocentesis/paracentesis if tense ascites/respiratory compromise due to ↑intra-abdominal pressure/↓renal perfusion; prophylactic LMWH (till onset of menses/end of first trimester if pregnancy), analgesia (oral/IV)—Acetaminophen or Paracetamol (PCM)/opiates (no NSAIDs), antiemetics, broad spectrum antibiotics if sepsis, surgery if ovarian torsion, rupture, or ectopic pregnancy.

PROGNOSIS

Self-limited, it regresses spontaneously, with normalization of Hct, ↓ascites and alleviation of clinical symptoms. If pregnancy occurs recovery may take longer, with ↑chances of preeclampsia and preterm delivery.

SUGGESTED READING

1. Prakash A, Mathur R. Ovarian hyperstimulation syndrome. Obstet Gynaecol. 2013;15:31-5.
2. RCOG Green Top Guideline No. 5 (2016). The management of hyperstimulation syndrome. [online] Available from https://www.rcog.org.uk/guidance/browse-all-guidance/green-top-guidelines/the-management-of-ovarian-hyperstimulation-syndrome-green-top-guideline-no-5/ [Last accessed September, 2024].

CHAPTER 41

Polycystic Ovarian Syndrome

DEFINITION

Heterogeneous, multisystem endocrinopathy in reproductive age women characterized by chronic anovulation resulting in infertility, irregular bleeding, obesity, hyperandrogenism, and metabolic disturbance [type 2 diabetes mellitus (DM), dyslipidemia, hypertension (HTN) and cardiovascular (CVS) disorder]; also, at ↑ risk of endometrial malignancy.

INCIDENCE

About 5–15%, increasing due to change in lifestyle, sedentary life diet and stress.

DIAGNOSTIC CRITERIA

Rotterdam criteria—two out of three should be present:

1. Anovulation/oligomenorrhea
2. Clinical and/or biochemical evidence of hyperandrogenism—hirsutism/acne/raised testosterone/androstenedione/dehydroepiandrosterone (DHEAS)
3. Polycystic ovaries—size >10 cc and >12 follicles of 2–9 mm in at least one ovary.

DIFFERENTIAL DIAGNOSIS

Adrenal and androgen producing ovarian tumor, hyperprolactinemia.

Irregular menses: Normal in the first-year postmenarche as part of pubertal transition.

- *>1 to <3 years postmenarche:* <21 or >45 days
- *>3 years postmenarche:* <21 or >35 days or <8 cycles per year
- *>1 year postmenarche:* >90 days for any one cycle

Obesity: 50–60%, centripetal, and Apple shape.

- *Phenotypes A/B/C/D:*
  - *Phenotype A:* Androgen excess + ovulatory dysfunction + polycystic ovarian morphology
  - *Phenotype B:* Androgen excess + ovulatory dysfunction
  - *Phenotype C:* Androgen excess + polycystic ovarian morphology
  - *Phenotype D:* Ovulatory dysfunction + polycystic ovarian morphology

PATHOPHYSIOLOGY (FLOWCHART 1)

Multifactorial involving endocrine, metabolic, genetic, epigenetic, and environmental factors. Familial occurrence identified with sex-linked mode of inheritance.

Enhanced serine phosphorylation unification activity in ovary (hyperandrogen) and reduced insulin receptor activity peripherally (insulin resistance).

- Obesity (↑ adipose tissue) → ↑ secretion of Leptin, adiponectin, and cytokines → interferes with insulin signaling path in liver and muscle → insulin resistance and hyperinsulinemia.
- Insulin resistance with resulting hyperinsulinemia initiates polycystic ovary syndrome (PCOS) in 50–70% cases.
- Raised luteinizing hormone (LH) level in response to increased insulin level causes infertility and miscarriage. It also causes increased production of androgen from ovaries.

Endocrine Changes in Polycystic Ovary Syndrome (Stein–Leventhal Syndrome)

- ↑ LH, FSH normal, LH/FSH ratio >2.5; mildly ↑ thyroid-stimulating hormone (TSH) and prolactin level; ± ↓ sex hormone binding globulin (SHBG); ↑testosterone and epiandrostenedione level rise; fasting blood glucose/fasting insulin ratio <4.5 suggest insulin resistance, ↑triglyceride, ↓ high-density lipoprotein (HDL); ↑ Anti-Müllerian hormone (AMH) level.
- Ultrasound and AMH should not be used for diagnosis in those within 8 years of menarche **(Flowchart 1)**.

Flowchart 1: Pathogenesis of polycystic ovarian syndrome.

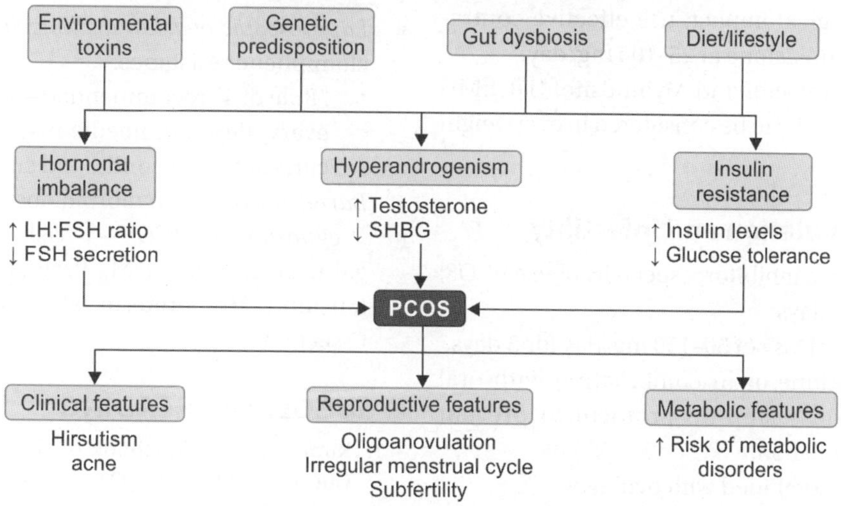

(FSH: follicle-stimulating hormone; LH: luteinizing hormone; PCOS: polycystic ovary syndrome; SHBG: sex hormone binding globulin)

MANAGEMENT

Women with PCOS may be seeking care for any one or more of the following:

- Menstrual abnormality
- Symptoms of androgen excess (hirsutism, acne, and alopecia)
- Infertility

Long-term health risks in women with PCOS include:

- Increased risk for endometrial hyperplasia and neoplasia
- Increased risk for infertility
- Increased risk for type 2 diabetes
- Increased risk for cardiovascular disease

Treatment—multidisciplinary involving reproductive endocrinologist, dermatologist, infertility specialist, psychiatrist, and dietician. Shared decision making.

Lifestyle Modification

- Exercise alone or multicomponent diet combined with exercise and behavioral strategies recommended for improving metabolic health.
- *Behavioral support:* SMART goals (Specific, Measurable, Achievable, Realistic and Timely).
- *Exercise:* 150–300 minutes of moderate intensity activities or 75–150 minutes of vigorous intensity exercise per week, plus muscle strengthening on 2 nonconsecutive days per week.
- Yoga and meditation
- Weight loss of even 5% in overweight and obese PCOS leads to significant clinical and endocrine improvement. Life-long focus on weight reduction.
- Adequate attention should be given to psychological symptom of anxiety, depression, and poor body image impacting overall quality of life.
- Counseling for long-term consequence of PCOS such as metabolic syndrome, type 2 diabetes, cardiovascular complications, sleep apnea, endometrial hyperplasia, and cancer.

PHARMACOLOGICAL TREATMENT

With Nonfertility Features

- *Combined oral contraceptive pills*—for irregular bleeding/hirsutism, not much difference between low dose or high dose preparation, used for 6–9 months, progestin-only pills can be used for endometrial protection.
- *Metformin*—In PCOS and body mass index (BMI) >25 kg/m^2 for anthropometric and metabolic outcomes, maximum dose is 2.5 g in adults and 2 g in adolescent, can be combined with combined oral contraceptives (COCs) for hirsutism in irregular menstrual bleeding.
- *Antiobesity agents*—Liraglutide, Semaglutide, and Orlistat can be considered in higher weight adults, effective contraception should be used.

- *Antiandrogen agents*—Treat hirsutism for allaying negative psychological impact, use effective contraception, and Spironolactone at 25–100 mg/day.
- *Inositol*—D-chiro-inositol and Myoinositol (DCI:MI) in combination of 40:1 can be considered in overweight PCOS.

Women with Anovulation and Infertility

- *Letrozole:* Aromatase inhibitor; especially obese PCOS; 2.5–5 mg/day for 5 days.
- *Clomiphene citrate:* Dose of 50–150 mg/day for 5 days.
- *Gonadotropins:* Alone or in combination with oral ovulogens; low dose step-up protocol to prevent ovarian hyperstimulation.
- Metformin can be combined with ovulogens.
- *In vitro fertilization:* Prefer antagonist protocol with agonist trigger and embryo freezing to prevent ovarian hyperstimulation.
- *Acne:* Eflornithine cream, mechanical treatment such as bleaching, waxing, plucking, electrolysis, laser therapy, reassurance, and support.

SURGICAL MANAGEMENT

- *Laparoscopic ovarian drilling:* Second line therapy in clomiphene resistance.
  - "Rule of 4" recommended—four punctures in each ovary, depth of needle insertion 4 mm, electrical current for 4 seconds, and current of 40 watts.
- *Bariatric surgery:* In morbid obese, BMI >40 kg/m^2
- *Pregnancy in PCOS*—↑ risk of abortion, weight gain, gestational DM, Pregnancy-induced hypertension (PIH), preterm labor, and increased rate of C-section.

SUGGESTED READING

1. Kumar. Shaw's Textbook of Gynaecology, 18th edition. Gurugram: Elsevier; 2022.
2. Taylor HS, Pal L, Seti E. Spernoff's Clinical Gynecologic Endocrinology and infertility, 9th edition. Gurugram: Wolters Kluwer; 2021.
3. Teede HJ, Tay CT, Laven JJE, Dokras A, Moran LJ, Piltonen TT, et al. International evidence-based guidelines for the assessment and management of polycystic ovary syndrome. J Clin Endocrinol Metab. 2023;108(10):2447-69.

NOTES

NOTES

SECTION 8

Urogynecology

Section Authors: *Jyoti Baghel, Babita Kumari, Saumya Agarwal*

CHAPTER 42

Vesicovaginal Fistulas

Obstetric fistulas are abnormal communication between female genital tract and urinary [most common—vesicovaginal fistula (VVF)]/gastrointestinal [most common—rectovesical fistula (RVF)] tract as a result of obstetric trauma, due to prolonged or obstructed labor leading to urinary/fecal incontinence. The VVF is an abnormal communication between urinary bladder and vagina.

Classification of vesicovaginal fistulas: Different classification systems based on etiology (congenital/acquired), site (Marion Sims), clinical findings (Goh—site, size, and scarring), surgical (anatomic/physiologic location with regard to surgical technique and results) (Waaldijk—continence mechanism), the World Health Organization (WHO) classification.

ACCORDING TO EXTENT OF INVOLVEMENT AND COMPLEXITY

Simple: Single, size ≤2 cm, does not involve ureter, no radiation exposure or malignancy, and vaginal length maintained normally.

Complicated: >1 in number, intermediate/large size, previous radiotherapy, associated with tumors in pelvic area, vagina shortened, ureteral or trigonal involvement, and failed previous repair.

ACCORDING TO THEIR SIZE AND SITE IN VAGINA

- High vaginal—proximally in vagina
- Low vaginal—distally in vagina
- Mid vaginal—centrally in vagina.

CAUSES

- Congenital genitourinary fistulas are rare, commonly associated with renal or urogenital anomalies.
- Most VVF are acquired and usually due to either obstetric injury or pelvic surgery.
- *In developing countries*: Obstetric trauma, commonly due to prolonged or obstructed labor or complicated C-section (CS) (>70% of VVF), due to ischemic pressure necrosis of soft tissues compressed between fetal head and maternal pelvic bone.
- *In developed countries,* iatrogenic injury at time of pelvic surgery (90% of VVF).
- *Other causes:* Radiation therapy, advanced pelvic cancers, and injuries in sexual assault.

SYMPTOMS

- Continuous leak of urine from vagina after recent delivery/surgery.
- Other less specific symptoms of genitourinary fistula include fever, pain, ileus, and bladder irritability.

DIAGNOSIS

- Detailed history and physical examination
- *On local examination:* Extra urethral leakage of urine, sodden and excoriated vulvar skin, and varying degree of perineal tears.
- Vaginal fluid creatinine content >17 mg/dL is consistent with urine.
- *On speculum examination:*
    - Size, site, and number of fistula.
    - In case of small fistula, only a puckered area is seen on anterior vaginal wall mucosa.
    - Complete perineal tear and recto vaginal fistula can be seen.
    - Metal catheter can be passed through the external urethral meatus into the bladder and if it comes out through the fistula, it confirms VVF.

THREE SWAB TEST "TAMPON TEST"

To differentiate between type of fistulas. "Three" cotton swabs are placed in vagina—at introitus, in middle and in anterior fornix. Methylene blue is instilled into bladder

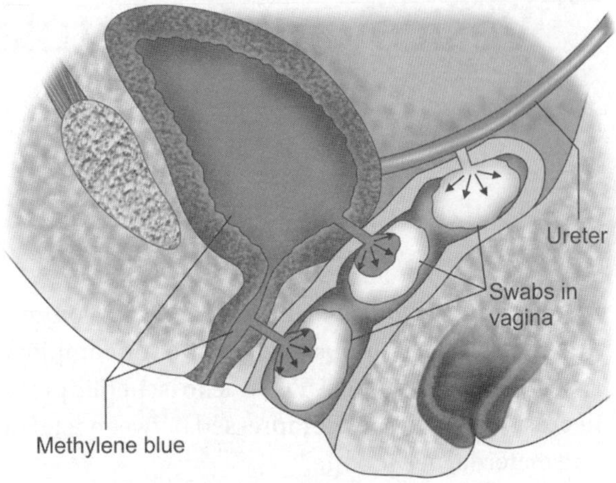

Fig. 1: Three swab test.
Source: Konar H. DC Dutta's Textbook of Gynecology, 8th edition. New Delhi: Jaypee Brothers Medical Publishers; 2020.

via rubber catheter. Patient is asked to walk for 5 minutes, then swabs are taken out.

Result:

- Top swab soaked, but unstained—ureterovaginal fistula
- Middle swab stained with dye—VVF
- Bottom swab stained with dye—urethrovaginal fistula

Figure 1 shows interpretation of three swab test.

INVESTIGATIONS

Urine routine and microscopy (R/M) and culture and sensitivity (C/S), high vaginal swabs (HVS)-C/S, full blood count (FBC) renal function test (RFT), transvaginal ultrasound (TVS).

Cystourethroscopy: Localizes site of fistula, its proximity to trigone/ureteral orifices, and determines viability of surrounding bladder mucosa.

Intravenous urogram (IVU)/computed tomography (CT) urogram to exclude coexistent ureteric injury or fistula (10% of VVFs associated with ureteric fistulas).

Ascending pyelography to supplement findings of intravenous pyelogram (IVP).

TREATMENT

Conservative treatment—In fistulas 1 cm in size or smaller: Spontaneous closure with continuous catheter drainage advised for 10–12 weeks along with antibiotics cover.

Surgical treatment: If no improvement >3 months of catheter or large in size, referral to specialist center with urosurgery facilities.

Timing of Repair

- Dictum is that best to repair the fistula at its first closure during index surgery.
- Obstetrical fistula 3 months after delivery.
- Surgical/gynecological fistula:
  - If recognized within 48 hours—can be repaired immediately as less inflammation and tissue is more viable.
  - If >48 hours, repair >10–12 weeks.
- Radiation induced fistula >12 months
- In failure of treatment reattempt >3 months
- Repair should be tension-free, water-tight, and uninfected.

Routes of Repair: Vaginal/Abdominal

- Vaginal route associated with ↓operative times, ↓blood loss, ↓morbidity, and ↓hospital stays.
- It also allows easy access for other necessary equipment, like ureteral stents especially if fistula is located near ureteral orifices.

Vaginal Approach

- Vaginal flap splitting
- *Latzko technique (most commonly used):* In this technique, vaginal epithelium is dissected from underlying fascia around fistula tract, followed by circumscribe incision around fistula which is closed with purse-string suture.

Abdominal approach: With this route, the fistula is accessed and excised through an intentional cystotomy. Suitable for: (1) Proximally situated fistula in narrow vagina, (2) closely located to ureteral orifices, (3) with coexisting ureteric fistula, (4) persists after prior repair attempts, (5) complex configuration, or (7) requires an abdominal inter position graft.

- Transvesical—through bladder
- Tansperitoneal—through peritoneal cavity
- Combined

Interposition flaps: Surrounding tissue vascularity is essential for successful genitourinary fistula repair healing. The omental J-flap, which is an abdominal option, whereas a Martius bulbospongiosus fat pad flap is used during vaginal procedures.

POSTOPERATIVE CARE

- Continuous drainage of bladder via catheter for 14–21 days.

- Hydration to ensure bladder irrigation and to prevent clots from obstructing bladder.
- Always check for catheter blockage and try to prevent it, so that no bladder distension or tension on suture lines.
- Suprapubic catheter for fistula.
- Cystogram to check bladder integrity before discontinuing the bladder drainage.

POSTOPERATIVE COMPLICATIONS

- *Early:*
  - ↑ bleeding
  - Surgical site infection
  - Urinary tract infection
  - Continuous urine leakage through fistula
- *Late:*
  - Abdominopelvic adhesions (abdominal route)
  - Dyspareunia and tenderness (vaginal route)
  - ↓vaginal length/shortening and stenosis (vaginal route)

SUGGESTED READING

1. Hoffman BL, Schorge JO, Halvorson LM, Hamid CA, Corton MM, Schaffer JI. Williams Gynecology, 4th edition. United States: McGraw-Hill Education; 2020.
2. Konar H. DC Dutta's Textbook of Gynecology, 8th edition. New Delhi: Jaypee Brothers Medical Publishers; 2020.

CHAPTER 43

Vault Prolapse

DEFINITION

Descent of the apex of vaginal vault or cuff scar [point C on the pelvic organ prolapse quantification (POP-Q) system] after hysterectomy.

INCIDENCE

- 11.6% in hysterectomies done for prolapse.
- 1.8% in hysterectomies done for other benign diseases.

DIAGNOSIS AND INVESTIGATIONS

- POP-Q classification is used to assess vault prolapse clinically. Also, it helps in site-directed repair, assessment of outcomes, and comparison of results postoperatively.
- Urodynamic assessment is not recommended routinely if no symptoms of stress urinary incontinence (SUI) is present.
- Can use quality of life assessment questionnaires.

MEASURES FOR PREVENTION OF VAULT PROLAPSE

- McCall culdoplasty at the time of vaginal hysterectomy (Both uterosacral ligaments are approximated by continuous sutures, to obliterate peritoneum of posterior cul-de-sac as high as possible).
- Suturing vaginal cuff to cardinal and uterosacral ligaments in both total abdominal hysterectomy (TAH), and vaginal hysterectomy (VH), and high circumferential obliteration of pouch of Douglas.
- Sacrospinous fixation (SSF) when the vault descends to the introitus during closure in vaginal hysterectomy [Failure if point C >two-thirds total vaginal length (TVL)—vaginal apex descending below upper one-third of vagina, or one of points Ba or Bp being >0 cm, i.e., anterior (Ba)/posterior (Bp) vaginal. Wall prolapsing beyond the hymen].

Subtotal hysterectomy is not recommended for prevention.

CLINICAL PRESENTATION

- Asymptomatic
- Symptoms of bulge and pressure below, sexual dysfunction, lower urinary tract dysfunction, or defecatory dysfunction.

MANAGEMENT: PELVIC FLOOR MULTIDISCIPLINARY TEAM

Conservative management:

- Pelvic floor muscle training for stage I–II vaginal prolapse.
- Vaginal pessaries for stage II–IV vaginal prolapse (counseling for sexual function, regular pessary changes, and possible complications—ulceration, vaginal bleeding, and risk of fistula).

Surgical Management (Only for *Symptomatic* Patients)

Aims postoperative POP-Q stage of I or O in apical compartment objectively, but primarily restoration of normal vaginal anatomy, improvement in vaginal bulge symptoms, and restoration/maintenance of normal bladder, and bowel and sexual function.

- *Open abdominal sacrocolpoplexy (ASC):* Involves apical suspension of the vault with a permanent mesh (attached to anterior and posterior aspect of vault) fixed to the anterior longitudinal ligament of the sacrum. Failure in one-third, mesh erosion was observed in 2–11%, bowel injury, sacral myelitis, and severe bleeding due to trauma to blood vessels (venous sinuses) overlying anterior longitudinal ligament. Lower rates of dyspareunia, recurrent vault prolapse, and postoperative SUI as compared to SSF.
- *Sacrospinous fixation:* Unilateral anchoring of the vaginal vault to the sacrospinous ligament using either absorbable or nonabsorbable sutures. Earlier recovery as compared to ASC. But high incidence of postoperative anterior compartment prolapses and SUI, buttock

pain, pudendal nerve injury, temporary irritation of sciatic nerve, and partial ureteral obstruction rarely. Not appropriate in women with short vaginal length and preexisting dyspareunia (ASC better).

- *Laparoscopic and robotic sacrocolpopexy (LSC and RSC):* In selected women with primary vault prolapse.
- *High uterosacral ligament suspension (HUSLS):* May be done vaginally, abdominally, or laparoscopically and involves bilateral suspension of the vaginal vault to the uterosacral ligaments near the level of the ischial spine. There is a high risk of ureteric injury, so it is offered only in context of research or audit.
- *Colpocleisis:* It is closure of vagina using purse-string closure technique. Done in frail, elderly women (not fit for surgery) or women who do not want to retain sexual function.
- *Concomitant **occult** SUI:* Colposuspension can be done along with sacrocolpopexy.
- *Concomitant **overt** SUI:* Mid urethral tape may be used when vaginal surgical approaches are done. Colposuspension with sacrocolpopexy is not effective in overt SUI.
- No role of transvaginal mesh or permanent sutures, due to risk of erosion.

SUGGESTED READING

1. Green-top Guideline No. 46. (2015). Posthysterectomy vaginal vault prolapse. [online] Available from https://www.rcog.org.uk/guidance/browse-all-guidance/green-top-guidelines/post-hysterectomy-vaginal-vault-prolapse-green-top-guideline-no-46/ [Last accessed September, 2024].

NOTES

SECTION 9

Premalignant and Malignant Lesions

Section Authors: *Manoj Kumar Tangri, Babita Kumari, Chanchal Choudhary*

CHAPTER 44

Cervical Intraepithelial Neoplasia

INTRODUCTION

Screening for premalignant lesion of cancer (Ca) cervix is successful in reducing Ca cervix by 79% and reducing mortality by 70%.

TECHNIQUES

Conventional papanicolaou (PAP)/liquid-based cytology (LBC)/automated image-guided slide screening system/ high-risk human papillomavirus (hrHPV) deoxyribonucleic acid (DNA). Limited resource setting—visual inspection with acetic acid (VIA) via 5% acetic acid.

SCREENING OPTIONS

At present three options for cervical cancer screening in individuals aged 30–65 years:

1. Primary hrHPV testing every 5 years
2. Cervical cytology alone every 3 years
3. Cotesting with a combination of cytology + hrHPV every 5 years.

- *HPV infection*—Primary cause of cervical intraepithelial neoplasia (CIN) and Ca cervix. HPV DNA gets integrated into host DNA for reproduction, causing malignant transformation, by E6 and E7 HPV oncoprotein.
- Most of CIN—HPV can be detected.
- 90% of HPV infections are associated with CIN.
- High-risk HPV types 16, 18, 31, 33, 35, 39, 45, 51, 52, 56, 58, 59, and 68.
- HPV 16 most **common** type associated with invasive Ca and CIN2, CIN3.
- HPV 18 >16 **specific** for invasive Ca.
- *HPV testing*—Molecular target for testing—DNA, E6/E7, messenger ribonucleic acid (mRNA)
- Cotesting—cervical smear + HPV.

FOGSI (FEDERATION OF OBSTETRIC AND GYNAECOLOGICAL SOCIETIES OF INDIA) CRITERIA OF VARIOUS SINGLE VISIT APPROACH STRATEGIES (TABLES 1 TO 3)

See and Treat

- In colposcopy clinics
- Patient referred with abnormal cytology report.
- Colposcopy scoring indicates a high-grade lesion.
- Simultaneous treatment done—excision or ablation.
- Low probability of overtreatment because of high specificity of cytology.
- Posthoc analysis of biopsy report/excision specimen.

Screen and Treat

- In public health programs
- VIA detects abnormal lesion
- Criteria for ablation fulfilled
- Treat immediately, with or without biopsy
- Lower probability of overtreatment in high prevalence areas
- Posthoc analysis is possible if biopsy taken

Eligibility for See-and-Treat Excision Procedures

- Lesion should be entirely visible limited to cervix.
- Entire lesion should be located on ectocervix without any vaginal and/or endocervical extension.
- There is no suspicion of invasive cancer.
- Not pregnant

Tables 1 to 3: Federation of Obstetric and Gynaecological Societies of India (FOGSI)—Resource-based Strategies for Cervical Cancer Screening and Management of CIN.

Table 4 displays United States Preventive Services Task Force recommendations for routine cervical screening.

TABLE 1: FOGSI resource-based strategies for screening and management of CIN.

Setting	*Screening tools*	*Triage tools*	*Management options*	*Single visit approach*
Good resource setting	• Primary HPV test or • Cotesting • (HPV test + cytology) or • Cytology or • VIA	• Cytology + newer modalities • HPV test • HPV genotyping-16/18 • colposcopy and biopsy** • VIA and biopsy	• LEEP • Conization • Cryotherapy • Thermal coagulation	See and treat approach
Limited resource settings[#]	VIA HPV[#]	Colposcopy, if available biopsy**	• Cryotherapy • LEEP • Conization • Thermal coagulation	• Screen and treat • Screen, see, and treat approach

[#]Newer modalities [p16, Ki 67, messenger ribonucleic acid (mRNA) testing, E6, E7 protein testing].

** Biopsy from any abnormal areas.

(CIN: cervical intraepithelial neoplasia; FOGSI: Federation of Obstetric and Gynaecological Societies of India; HPV: human papillomavirus; LEEP: loop electrosurgical excision procedure; VIA: visual inspection with acetic acid)

TABLE 2: FOGSI resource-based modalities for screening and management of CIN.

	Good-resource settings	*Limited-resource settings*
Modalities	• HPV testing – Primary HPV testing – Cotesting (HPV and cytology) • Cytology • VIA	VIA (Affordable HPV testing may be introduced if feasible)
Target age group (years)	25–65	30–65 (N.B.: In postmenopausal women, screening with VIA may not be as effective)
Age to start (years)	Cytology at 25 primary HPV testing/ cotesting at 30	VIA at 30
Frequency	Primary HPV testing or cotesting—every 5 years cytology every 3 years	Every 5 years (at least 1–3 times in a lifetime)

(CIN: cervical intraepithelial neoplasia; FOGSI: Federation of Obstetric and Gynaecological Societies of India; HPV: human papillomavirus; VIA: visual inspection with acetic acid)

Eligibility for Screen-and-Treat (Ablative Procedures)

- Lesion should be entirely visible and occupy not more than two quadrants of cervix.
- Entire lesion should be located on ectocervix without any vaginal and/or endocervical extension.
- Lesion can be adequately covered by largest cryotherapy probe available.
- There is no suspicion of invasive cancer.
- Screen-and-treat by cryotherapy is contraindicated in cases of postcoital or postmenopausal bleeding, obvious cervical growth, irregular surface, or bleeds on touch.

MANAGEMENT

- CIN1—60–85% regress, yearly co-testing. On 12 month follow-up if negative then further management according to age-appropriate screening.
- CIN1 persisting for >24 months, then colposcopic/ thermal ablation.
- CIN1—atypical squamous cells (ASC)-H—high-grade squamous intraepithelial lesion (HSIL)—consider loop excision.
- CIN2, CIN3—Neoplastic precursors, loop electrosurgical excision procedure (LEEP) preferred treatment, and ablative therapy **not** recommended.

TABLE 3: FOGSI resource-based follow-up for screening and management of CIN.

	Good-resource settings	*Limited-resource settings*
Age to stop (years)	• 65 with consistent negative results in last 15 years • Women with no prior screening should undergo tests once at 65 years and, if negative, they should exit screening	
Follow-up method after treatment; interval	HPV testing (preferred) or cytology 12 months	VIA 12 months
Screening following abnormal reports >CIN2+, irrespective of method of treatment	20 years	
Screening in hysterectomized women	• *Following hysterectomy in which cervix was removed for benign causes:* No need for screening, unless there is history of previous cervical intraepithelial neoplasia (CIN) • Absence of cervix must be confirmed by clinical records or examination • If indications for hysterectomy unclear, screening may be performed at clinician's discretion	
Follow-up in women with CIN in hysterectomy HPE report	Need to be screened with HPV at 6 months and 18 months	
Screening of immunocompromised women	• Start within 1 year of initiation of sexual activity • HPV testing/cotesting/cytology/VIA • Every 2–3 years	• VIA/(affordable HPV testing if available) • Every 3 years (at least twice as often as general population)

(CIN: cervical intraepithelial neoplasia; FOGSI: Federation of Obstetric and Gynaecological Societies of India; HPE: histopathology; HPV: human papillomavirus; VIA: visual inspection with acetic acid)

TABLE 4: USPSTF recommendations.

Population	*Recommendation*	*USPSTF recommendation grade*
Aged <21 years	No screening	D
Aged 21–29 years	Cytology alone every 3 years	A
Aged 30–65 years	*Any one of the following:* • Cytology alone every 3 years • FDA-approved primary hrHPV testing alone every 5 years • Cotesting (hrHPV testing and cytology) every 5 years	A
Aged >65 years	No screening after adequate negative prior screening results	D
Hysterectomy with removal of the cervix	No screening in individuals who do not have a history of high-grade cervical precancerous lesions or cervical cancer	D

(FDA: Food and Drug Administration; hrHPV: high-risk human papillomavirus; USPSTF: United States Preventive Services Task Force)

TREATMENT OPTIONS

- *Loop electrosurgical excision*—Tissue effect depends on—number of electrons (size of wire), power (watts), water content of tissue. Low power and large wire—electrocautery effect—large tissue damage. High power and small wire loop—electrosurgical effect. Cutting due to steam. Used as treatment in HSIL. Side-effects—preterm labor, preterm premature rupture of membranes (PPROM), and low birth weight (LBW) babies.
- *Cryotherapy*—surface epithelium of cervix is destroyed by crystallizing intracellular water. The temperature required is –20 to –30°, done by nitrous oxide, carbon dioxide. In freeze-thaw-freeze method, ice-ball achieved 5 mm beyond the edge of the probe. Time taken for procedure = pressure achieved, relatively safe. Side-effects—infection, cervical stenosis (rarely), failure—CIN3, lesion in endocervix.
- *Thermal ablation*—Probe heated to 100°, applied for 20–40 seconds, epithelial and stromal destruction. Multiple applications required. Prerequisites for cryo/thermal ablation—(1) entire lesion visible/ transformation zone is of type 1/2 where probe tip can

reach the upper limit; (2) No suspicion of invasive/glandular disease.

- *Conization*—Diagnostic as well as therapeutic, indicated for CIN3, atypical glandular cells (AGC), and adenocarcinoma in situ (AIS). It is also used in conditions: (1) Squamo-columnar junction not evaluable through colposcopy; (2) limits of lesion cannot be viewed by colposcopy; (3) Endocervical curettage (ECC) positive for CIN 2/3. (4) Microinvasion suspected; (5) colposcopy unable to rule out invasive cancers; and (6) lack of correlation between cytology, HPV, biopsy, and colposcopy results.
- *Hysterectomy*:
  - Recurrent high-grade CIN
  - Evidence of microinvasion
  - Co-occurring gynecological diseases such as fibroid, endometriosis, and pelvic inflammatory disease (PID).

SUGGESTED READING

1. ACOG Practice Advisory. (2020). Updated Guidelines for Management of Cervical Cancer Screening Abnormalities. [online] Available from https://www.acog.org/clinical/clinical-guidance/practice-advisory/articles/2020/10/updated-guidelines-for-management-of-cervical-cancer-screening-abnormalities [Last accessed September, 2024].
2. ACOG Practice Advisory. (2021). Updated Cervical Cancer Screening Guidelines. [online] Available from https://www.acog.org/clinical/clinical-guidance/practice-advisory/articles/2021/04/updated-cervical-cancer-screening-guidelines [Last accessed September, 2024].
3. FOGSI Gynaecologic Oncology Committee. (2018). FOGSI GCPR Screening and Management of Preinvasive Lesions of Cervix and HPV Vaccination. [online] Available from https://www.fogsi.org/wp-content/uploads/2018/01/fogsi-gcpr-smplc-cervix-hpv-vaccination-document-2017-2018.pdf [Last accessed September, 2024].

CHAPTER 45

Cervical Cancer

DISEASE LOAD: GLOBALLY

- 662,301 new cases of cervical cancer were detected in 2022.
- 348,874 deaths were attributed to this malignancy.

In India

- Cervical cancer accounted 9.0% (127,526) of new cases in 2022.
- Mortality figures—79,906 deaths.

HUMAN PAPILLOMAVIRUS (TABLE 1)

Necessary precursor of precancer and cervical cancer.

Human Papillomavirus 16

It is the *most common human papillomavirus* (HPV) type *(50–60%)* in invasive cervical cancer.

Human Papillomavirus 18

- It is the second most common *(20–25%)* HPV type in invasive cervical cancer.
- Associated with cervical adenocarcinomas.

RISK FACTORS

- Having first sexual intercourse at an early age.
- Having many sexual partners.
- Giving birth to three or more children.
- Smoking cigarettes (this produces chemicals that can damage cervical cells).

TABLE 1: Classification of human papillomavirus (HPV) types based on cervical cancer risk.

High-risk	16, 18, 31, 33, 35, 39, 45, 51, 52, 56, 58, 59, 68, 73, 82
Probable high-risk	25, 53, 56
Low-risk	6, 11, 40, 42, 43, 44, 54, 61, 70, 72, 81

- Using oral contraceptives.
- Being infected with the human immunodeficiency virus (HIV), virus causing acquired immunodeficiency syndrome (AIDS).

DIAGNOSIS: CLINICAL PRESENTATION

- Postcoital or abnormal vaginal bleeding
- Malodorous vaginal discharge
- Symptoms such as persistent pain in the back, legs, or pelvis
- Weight loss, fatigue, and loss of appetite
- Vaginal discomfort
- Swelling in the legs
- In early stages, it is commonly asymptomatic.
- Gold-standard:
  - *Histopathological examination of cervical biopsy:* Direct biopsy or cone biopsy (conization) or endocervical curettage for endocervical lesions.
  - During colposcopy, the *endocervical curettage* method can lead to up to 75% false-negative results; thus, the positive results should be considered, and a negative result does not exclude the possibility of cancer.
- If lesion is visible—direct biopsy
- *If lesion not visible:* Colposcopy and biopsies of suspicious areas [if patients have abnormal cytology, and/or positive results for deoxyribonucleic acid (DNA)-HPV]
- The triad of clinical assessment, cytology, and colposcopy are the paths for diagnosis.
- Conization—*Cone biopsy* recommended *when* it is not possible to estimate stromal invasion through colposcopy and direct biopsy, or *when* colposcopy is unsatisfactory, or *when* cytopathological evaluation shows an intraepithelial high-grade lesion, or *when* there is a disagreement regarding methods for a suspect lesion.

HISTOPATHOLOGY

Types as per the World Health Organization (WHO) classification of female genital tumors:

- Squamous epithelial tumors:
  - Squamous cell carcinoma, HPV-associated
  - Squamous cell carcinoma, HPV-independent
  - Squamous cell carcinoma not otherwise specified (NOS)
- Glandular tumors:
  - Adenocarcinoma NOS
  - Adenocarcinoma, HPV-associated
  - Adenocarcinoma, HPV-independent
  - Gastric type
  - Adenocarcinoma, HPV-independent, clear cell type
  - Adenocarcinoma, HPV-independent, mesonephric type
  - Adenocarcinoma, HPV-independent, NOS
  - Endometrioid adenocarcinoma NOS
  - Carcinosarcoma NOS
  - Adenosquamous carcinoma
  - Mucoepidermoid carcinoma
  - Adenoid basal carcinoma
  - Carcinoma, undifferentiated, NOS
- Mixed epithelial and mesenchymal tumors—Adenosarcoma
- Germ cell tumors:
  - Endodermal sinus tumor
  - Yolk sac tumor NOS
  - Choriocarcinoma NOS

INTERNATIONAL FEDERATION OF GYNECOLOGY AND OBSTETRICS (FIGO) STAGING OF CANCER OF THE CERVIX UTERI (2018)

Stage I

Strictly confined to cervix (extension to uterine corpus disregarded):

- IA—Invasive carcinoma only by microscopy, maximum depth of invasion ≤5 mm
  - IA1 measured stromal invasion ≤3 mm in depth
  - IA2 measured stromal invasion >3 and ≤5 mm in depth
- IB—Invasive carcinoma with deepest invasion >5 mm (>Stage IA)
  - IB1—>5 mm depth of stromal invasion and ≤2 cm in greatest dimension
  - IB2—>2 and ≤4 cm in greatest dimension
  - IB3—>4 cm in greatest dimension

Stage II

Carcinoma spreads beyond uterus, but not to lower one-third of vagina or to pelvic wall.

- IIA—Limited to upper two-thirds of vagina without parametrial involvement:
  - IIA1 invasive carcinoma ≤4 cm in greatest dimension
  - IIA2 invasive carcinoma >4 cm in greatest dimension
- IIB—Parametrial involvement but not up to lateral pelvic wall.

Stage III

- Carcinoma involves lower one-third of vagina and/or extends to pelvic wall and/or causes hydronephrosis or nonfunctioning kidney and/or involves pelvic and/or para-aortic lymph nodes
- IIIA—Spreads to lower one-third of vagina, with no extension to lateral pelvic wall.
- IIIB—Extension to pelvic wall and/or hydronephrosis or nonfunctioning kidney.
- IIIC—Involvement of pelvic and/or para-aortic lymph nodes.
  - IIIC1—Pelvic lymph node metastasis only
  - IIIC2—Para-aortic lymph node metastasis

Stage IV

Carcinoma spreads beyond true pelvis or has involved (biopsy proven) mucosa of bladder or rectum. A bullous edema, as such, does not permit a case to be allotted to stage IV.

- IVA—Spread of the growth to adjacent pelvic organs.
- IVB—Spread to distant organs.

IMAGING AND PATHOLOGY

Supplement clinical findings with respect to tumor size and extent, in all stages.

Adding notation of r (imaging) and p (pathology) to indicate findings that are used to allocate to stage IIIC. For example, if imaging indicates pelvic lymph node metastasis, the stage allocation would be stage IIIC1r; if confirmed by pathological findings, it would be stage IIIC1p.

- Staging based only on clinical findings—reliable just for patients placed in the extremes, such as IIIA, IIIB, or IVA.
- Magnetic resonance imaging (MRI)—Best method for primary tumor assessment.
- Positron emission tomography (PET) scan—Best option for lymph node evaluation.

Pathologic staging when surgical specimen is available—precise method to assess extent of disease. Staging should be established at diagnosis and not altered even at recurrence.

EARLY CANCER CERVIX: TREATMENT

- *Treatment options:* From IB to IIA, similar oncological outcomes with surgery or radiation therapy (RT) both.
- Surgery preferred primary mode of treatment in young, due to quality-of-life (QoL) issues, preserves ovarian and sexual function, and treats cancers that are likely to be radioresistant.
- Specimen available for pathology.
- Standard surgery is radical hysterectomy (RH) **(Table 2)** with bilateral pelvic lymph node dissection (BPLND).
- Fertility sparing surgery (radical trachelectomy)—may be considered based on appropriate stage, tumor size, and lymph-vascular space invasion (LVSI).
- Radiotherapy with/without chemo preferred in elderly, comorbidities, or poor functional status.

MICROINVASIVE CARCINOMA CERVIX (IA1/IA2): SURGERY

- *FIGO stage IA1:*
  - Conization enough, if no LVSI/type 1 hysterectomy
  - If LVSI +, type-1 extrafascial hysterectomy with BPLND
  - *Fertility sparing surgery:* Conization with close follow-up
- *FIGO stage IA2:*
  - Type 2 or type "B" RH with BPLND/sentinel lymph node (SLN)
  - *Fertility sparing surgery:* Conization with BPLND [open/minimally invasive surgery (MIS)]
  - Radical trachelectomy with BPLND (vaginal/abdominal/MIS)

TABLE 2: Types of radical hysterectomy.

	Simple extrafascial hysterectomy	*Modified radical hysterectomy*	*Radical hysterectomy (RH)*
Piver and Rutledge classification	Type I	Type II	Type III
Querleu–Morrow classification	Type A	Type B	Type C
Indication	Stage IA1	Type IA1 with LVSI IA2	Stage IB1 and IB2. Selected stage IIA
Uterus and cervix	Removed	Removed	Removed
Ovaries	Optional removal	Optional removal	Optional removal
Vaginal margin	None	1–2 cm	Upper one-quarter to one-third
Ureters	Not mobilized	Tunnel through broad ligament	Tunnel through broad ligament
Cardinal ligaments	Divided at uterine and cervical border	Divided where ureter transits broad ligaments	Divided at pelvic side wall
Uterosacral ligaments	Divided at cervical border	Partially removed	Divided near sacral origin
Urinary bladder	Mobilized to base of bladder	Mobilized to upper vagina	Mobilized to middle vagina
Rectum	Not mobilized	Mobilized below cervix	Mobilized below cervix
Surgical approach	Laparotomy or laparoscopy or robotic surgery	Laparotomy or laparoscopy or robotic surgery	Laparotomy or laparoscopy or robotic surgery

(LVSI: lymph-vascular space invasion)

INVASIVE CARCINOMA CERVIX (IB1, IB2, AND IIA1): SURGERY

- *FIGO stage IB1:* Low risk if, stromal invasion <50% and no lymph nodes on imaging: Type C1 radical hysterectomy with BPLND
- *Fertility sparing surgery in IA2 and IB1:* Radical trachelectomy with BPLND
- *FIGO stage IB2 and IIA1:* Type C radical hysterectomy with BPLND

TRACHELECTOMY

≤40 years, intends to have children, fertile patient, stage IA1 with LVSI or IA2 and IB1 stages (tumor <2 cm) with MRI showing no parametrial invasion or metastases to LN. Cervix with parametrium removed followed by anastomosis of the uterus with the vaginal end (+ Shirodkar cerclage). It can be done by open abdominal, vaginal, or by minimally invasive routes. When a vaginal approach is planned, the pelvic nodes are first removed laparoscopically and sent for frozen section to confirm node negativity, then proceed with radical trachelectomy vaginally. Alternatively, the nodes may first be assessed by conventional pathological methods and the radical trachelectomy done as a second surgery after 1 week.

MORBIDITY FROM STANDARD RADICAL HYSTERECTOMY (COMPLICATIONS)

Short-term

- Major hemorrhage
- Infection [urinary tract infections (UTIs) 20%]
- Damage to bladder, bowel ureters, ureteric/vesico fistula
- Injury to nerves (genitofemoral/obturator) up to 10%

Long-term

- Loss of fertility
- *Physical:*
  - Bowel, bladder, and sexual dysfunction
  - Lymphedema (10%)
  - Thigh pain
- Psychological, relationships, and cancer survivorship

Minimally invasive radical hysterectomy (MIS) associated with higher rate of recurrence than open approach in early-stage cervical cancer, but no difference in QoL between patients who had open and minimally invasive radical hysterectomy for early-stage cervical cancer.

TABLE 3: Sedlis intermediate risk factors criteria.*

Lymphovascular space invasion	*Stromal invasion*	*Tumor size (cm)*†
+	Deep third	Any
+	Middle third	≥2
+	Superficial third	≥5
–	Middle or deep third	≥4

*Criteria apply to node—negative, margin-negative, and parametria-negative cases.

†Size is determined by clinical palpation.

CERVICAL CANCER: RISK FACTORS

High Risk Factors (Peters Criteria): Any One or More

- *Parametrial invasion +ve*
- *Lymph nodes (Micro or macro metastasis) +ve*
- *Surgical margins +ve*

Table 3 shows Sedlis intermediate risk factors criteria.

Low Risk Factors

Nonspecific, size <2 cm, depth of invasion <10 mm, no LVSI and LN-ve.

- European Society for Medical Oncology clinical practice guidelines recommend that with intermediate risk no need for further adjuvant therapy (evidence level IIB).
- The FIGO CC recommends that postoperative radiotherapy required, but chemotherapy is not recommended, if a patient exhibits any two of the following risk factors: Tumor size >4 cm, LVSI, and deep SI.

INVASIVE CARCINOMA CERVIX (FIGO IA, IB1, IB2, AND IIA1): RADIATION

- Intracavitary brachytherapy (ICRT) alone:
  - Microinvasive disease
  - Small IB1 (<1 cm), especially if external beam radiotherapy (EBRT) relatively contraindicated
- Concurrent chemoradiotherapy (CCRT)—standard radiotherapy.

FIELD DESIGN FOR THE PELVIC RADIOTHERAPY

Table 4 shows the field design for the pelvic radiotherapy.

TABLE 4: Field design for the pelvic radiotherapy.

Field	Border	Landmark
AP-PA fields	Superior	L4–5 vertebral interspace
		2 cm below obturator foramen/3 cm
		Inferior to distal disease, whichever lower
Lateral fields	Lateral	1.5–2 cm lateral to the pelvic brim
	Superior	Same as AP-PA field
	Inferior	Same as AP-PA field
	Anterior	Anterior to the pubic symphysis
	Posterior	0.5 cm posterior to anterior border of S 2/3
		Vertebral junction, may include entire sacrum to cover the disease extent

(AP: anterior-posterior; PA: posterior-anterior)

INVASIVE CARCINOMA CERVIX (FIGO IIB-IVA): RADIATION ONLY

The CCRT is considered the standard treatment for patients with locally advanced cervical cancer.

Once-weekly infusion of Cisplatin (40 mg/m^2 weekly with appropriate hydration) for 5–6 cycles during external beam therapy is a commonly used concurrent chemotherapy regimen. If unable to receive Platinum chemotherapy, 5-Fluorouracil-based regimens are an acceptable alternative.

Combination of EBRT **(Table 4)** and ICRT maximizes the likelihood of locoregional control while minimizing the risk of treatment complications. The primary goal of EBRT is to sterilize local disease and to shrink the tumor to facilitate subsequent ICRT.

FIGO STAGE IVB/DISTANT METASTASES

Presentation with distant metastatic disease is rare, reported in about 2% of cases. Concurrent chemoradiation may have a better response than systemic chemotherapy with overall disease-free survivals of 69% and 57%, respectively, reported in patients with positive para-aortic and supraclavicular lymph nodes.

Currently, there is no role for prophylactic extended field radiotherapy (EFRT) in locally advanced cervical cancer. When para-aortic nodes are involved, EFRT with concurrent chemotherapy should be used.

POST-TREATMENT FOLLOW-UP

- Every 3–4 months for first 2–3 years
- Every 6 months till 5 years
- Annually for life

SUGGESTED READING

1. International Agency for Research on Cancer. (2022). Globocan. [online] Available from https://gco.iarc.fr/ [Last accessed September, 2024].

CHAPTER 46

Endometrial Hyperplasia

INTRODUCTION

Endometrial hyperplasia (EH) is defined as irregular proliferation of the endometrial glands with an increase in the gland to stroma ratio when compared with proliferative endometrium. Incidence of EH is estimated to be at least three times higher than endometrial cancer and if left untreated it can progress to endometrial cancer (EC).

RISK FACTORS

- Unopposed estrogen
- Increased body mass index (BMI)
- Anovulation [polycystic ovary syndrome (PCOS)/ Perimenopause]
- Estrogen secreting ovarian tumors [Granulosa cell tumor (GCT)]
- Drug-induced, e.g., prolonged use of Tamoxifen or estrogen-only hormone replacement therapy (HRT)

CLINICAL FEATURES

Symptoms

Abnormal uterine bleeding (AUB) includes heavy menstrual bleeding (HMB), intermenstrual bleeding (IMB), irregular bleeding, unscheduled bleeding on HRT, and postmenopausal bleeding (PMB).

Classification Systems for Endometrial Hyperplasia [Revised 2014 World Health Organization (WHO)]

- Hyperplasia without atypia
- Atypical hyperplasia

DIAGNOSTIC AND SURVEILLANCE METHODS

- Transvaginal ultrasonography
- Outpatient endometrial sampling
- Hysteroscopy-guided endometrial biopsy (especially if associated with polyp or other discrete focal lesion).
- *Diagnostic hysteroscopy and biopsy:* If outpatient sampling fails or is nondiagnostic.
- *Computed tomography (CT) and magnetic resonance imaging (MRI) or biomarkers:* Not recommended routinely.

MANAGEMENT

Endometrial Hyperplasia without Atypia

Majority of cases of EH without atypia will regress spontaneously during follow-up. Risk of progression to EC is <5% in 20 years.

Address the risk factors such as obesity and use of HRT.

Progestogen treatment is indicated in women who fail to regress following observation alone and in symptomatic women with abnormal uterine bleeding.

First-line treatment is Levonorgestrel-releasing intrauterine system (LNG-IUS). Those who decline LNG-IUS can be given continuous progestogens (Medroxyprogesterone 10–20 mg/day or Norethisterone 10–15 mg/day) for 6 months.

Endometrial surveillance: 6 monthly by endometrial biopsy. When two consecutive 6 monthly biopsies are negative patient can be discharged from follow-up. But long-term annual follow-up in those at high risk of relapse like BMI ≥35 kg/m^2 or those treated with oral progestogens.

If EH persists for 12 months despite treatment, the risk of underlying cancer is high and the chances of disease regression are low, such that hysterectomy is advised.

Hysterectomy indicated only in women not wanting to preserve their fertility when:

- Progression to atypical hyperplasia occurs during follow-up.
- There is no histological regression of hyperplasia despite 12 months of treatment.

- There is relapse of EH after completing progestogen treatment.
- There is persistence of bleeding symptom AUB.
- The woman declines to undergo endometrial surveillance or comply with medical treatment.

Postmenopausal women requiring surgical management for EH without atypia should be offered a bilateral salpingo-oophorectomy together with the total hysterectomy.

Atypical Endometrial Hyperplasia

Risk of progression to EC is ~29% at 20 years, and in ~43% concomitant endometrial cancer was found to be present, risk of coexisting ovarian cancer is 4%.

Laparoscopic total hysterectomy with bilateral salpingo-oophorectomy in postmenopausal women and in premenopausal women hysterectomy with bilateral salpingectomy is preferred. Removal of ovaries is decided on individual basis in premenopausal women.

Do **not** send frozen section analysis of the endometrium or do routine lymphadenectomy.

Women with Atypical Hyperplasia Who Wish to Preserve Their Fertility

Counsel about the risks of malignancy. Investigations prior to fertility-sparing treatment include tumor markers such as CA125 and imaging with transvaginal ultrasound (TVS) and/or MRI scan to rule out coexisting ovarian cancer and invasive endometrial cancer.

LNG-IUS is first-line or oral progestogens as second-line alternative.

When fertility is no longer required, offer hysterectomy.

Follow-up for these women: 3 monthly endometrial biopsies. Disease regression should be present in at least one biopsy sample before attempting to conceive, assisted reproductive technology (ART) preferred than waiting for spontaneous conception. Hysterectomy should be recommended to women with atypical EH once fertility is no longer required due to high relapse rate of disease and potential for disease progression. Also, if there is failure of regression of atypical hyperplasia by 12 months or there is evidence of progression to cancer, hysterectomy is recommended.

In asymptomatic women, after two consecutive negative biopsies, follow-up every 6–12 months until hysterectomy performed.

Hormone replacement therapy and endometrial hyperplasia: In those underwent hysterectomy, systemic estrogen-only HRT is recommended. Those who wish to continue (with EH) continuous combined HRT recommended especially with LNG-IUS as progesterone component.

Women on Tamoxifen for breast cancer treatment: Counseling about risk of developing EH and EC, promptly report if AUB, then the need for Tamoxifen should be reassessed and management should be according to histological type. LNG-IUS not recommended due to risk of recurrence of breast cancer in patients on Tamoxifen.

SUGGESTED READING

1. Green-top Guideline No. 67 RCOG/BSGE Joint Guideline. (2016). Management of Endometrial Hyperplasia. [online] Available from https://www.rcog.org.uk/guidance/browse-all-guidance/green-top-guidelines/management-of-endometrial-hyperplasia-green-top-guideline-no-67/ [Last accessed September, 2024].

CHAPTER 47

Borderline Ovarian Tumor

DEFINITION

Tumors of low malignant potential, that demonstrate higher proliferative activity compared with benign neoplasm, but no stromal invasion.

Incidence: About 10–15% of all epithelial ovarian neoplasm.

They typically occur in younger age group [cystic fibrosis (c.f.) invasive] and have excellent prognosis as they are usually diagnosed at an earlier stage. 5-year survival rate for stage 1 borderline ovarian tumor (BOT) varies from 95 to 97%.

RISK FACTORS

- Nulliparous women
- Young age

Lactation is protective. Oral contraceptive not proactive unlike invasive ovarian cancer.

Borderline ovarian tumors are low grade tumors and even if they progress to invasive disease, they tend to be low-grade invasive instead of high grade. Mutations of *BRAF/KRAS* pathway are commonly seen in BOT as compared to high-grade serous associated with *p53* mutation.

HISTOLOGICAL CLASSIFICATION

Stratified epithelium with nuclear atypia and ↑mitotic activity, and no stromal invasion. These are bilateral in 30%, may be associated with extraovarian lesions called implants which can be invasive/noninvasive.

- Serous [mucinous carcinoma (MC)]—50%
  - Micropapillary
  - Microinvasive
- Mucinous—46%
  - Intestinal
  - Endocervical/Mullerian
- Endometrioid, clear cell, Brenner, and mixed—4%

DIAGNOSIS

As asymptomatic, mostly diagnosed on incidental/routine examination; symptomatics have prolonged duration as compared to invasive (short duration)—pelvic pain, bloating, dyspareunia, menstrual irregularities, and pressure symptoms such as frequency of micturition and constipation.

INVESTIGATIONS

- CA125, CA19-9, ultrasonography (USG) pelvis and color Doppler, and magnetic resonance imaging (MRI)
- Transvaginal ultrasound (TVS)—varies from unilocular cysts, minimally septate with papillary projections, markedly septate with plaque-like excrescences to solid lesions with exophytic papillary projections.

MANAGEMENT

Multidisciplinary team (MDT) including gynecologist, radiologist, pathologist, and specialist nurse. It should be individualized according to age, stage of disease, desire for pregnancy, and nature of peritoneal implants. Staging laparotomy and cytoreductive surgery with frozen section is standard treatment. If frozen section shows borderline, in older woman with no fertility concerns a complete staging includes:

- Exploration of entire abdominal cavity with peritoneal washings
- Total abdominal hysterectomy
- Bilateral salpingo-oophorectomy
- Infracolic omentectomy
- Appendicectomy in mucinous tumors.
- No role of lymphadenectomy unless invasive reported on frozen section.

ROLE OF RESTAGING AND COMPLETION SURGERY

Determined by three factors: (1) Histological subtype of BOT, (2) completeness of primary surgery, and (3) fertility desires.

Restaging may be done if associated with micropapillary type, invasive implants or deoxyribonucleic acid (DNA) aneuploidy. It includes—peritoneal washings, omentectomy, with exploration of peritoneal cavity with/without hysterectomy, and removal of contralateral ovary (no role of lymphadenectomy).

ROLE OF CONSERVATIVE SURGERY AND SUBSEQUENT FERTILITY

Counseling regarding risks of recurrence and need for follow-up. Complete staging with preservation of uterus and at least a part of one ovary, i.e., cystectomy or unilateral salpingo-oophorectomy, with/without infracolic omentectomy, and peritoneal washings. Systematic biopsies of macroscopically normal contralateral ovary not recommended.

Relapse rates are higher after cystectomy and salpingo-oophorectomy compared with radical surgery. But most recurrent disease is of borderline type, easily resectable and associated with excellent prognosis.

ROLE OF LAPAROSCOPY

Chances of cyst rupture, port site metastasis, and understaging leading to ↑risk of recurrence, so in absence of clear evidence, staging, and treatment of BOT should ideally be performed by midline laparotomy.

No role for adjuvant chemotherapy in BOTs treatment.

FOLLOW-UP

- Every 3 months for the first 2 years.
- Every 6 months for the next 2 years.
- Annually thereafter, by clinical examination and TVS.

SUGGESTED READING

1. Gershenson DM. Management of borderline ovarian tumours. Obstet Gynaecol. 2012;14:115-20.

NOTES

SECTION 10

Sexual and Reproductive Health

Section Authors: *Mridu Sinha, Jyoti Baghel, Saumya Agarwal*

CHAPTER 48

Sexual Assault

INTRODUCTION

Sexual assault occurs when: (1) A person intentionally touches another person; (2) the touching is sexual; and (3) the person does not consent. *Serious sexual assault*—when a person commits assault by penetration of vagina/anus of another person with a part of the body or anything else, without that person's consent. *Rape,* where penetration of the vagina, anus, or mouth of a person has occurred with a penis without consent.

Worldwide 35% of women experience physical and/or sexual intimate partner/nonpartner violence. 1:5 (16–59 years) in their lifetime, 1:20 experience serious form; 85%—domestic violence, 5%—rape, and 11%—sexual offences. 15% of assaults on individuals are under 12 years old. About 80–90% of offenders known to their victims and 20% has mental health problem [post-traumatic stress disorder (PTSD)].

VULNERABLE POPULATION

Young and poor, poor health; Social housing; Single, separated, or divorced; <16 years, mental health problem/ learning difficulties; Migrants and trafficking females in sex-industry; and transgender.

APPROACH

History Taking

A brief history of the assault should be recorded in clinical notes concentrating on what happened, when, where, and by whom to know scenario, and assist in deciding about sites for sexually transmitted infections (STI) swabs as well as the possible need for psychosocial support. Consent, confidentiality, and careful documentation in clinical notes is essential.

On examination (O/E)—Minor injuries that do not require suturing should not be cleaned initially because samples can be taken from these sites for deoxyribonucleic acid (DNA) evidence. Each injury should be described in the clinical notes, including the shape, depth, color, and tenderness; as well as the type of injury like—bruise, abrasion, or laceration; and their measurement and relation to bony points.

Needs after sexual assault are:

- *Immediate needs (within 7 days of assault)*—Immediate safety—treatment of injuries, baseline screening for STIs and/or prophylaxis for bacterial STIs with follow-up schedule. Baseline human immunodeficiency virus (HIV) test and HIV postexposure prophylaxis postsexual assault (PEPSE) within 72 hours. Hepatitis B vaccination ± hepatitis B immunoglobulin if assailant likely or known to be surface antigen carrier. Prevention of pregnancy. Referral for forensic medical examination (FME) to gather DNA evidence and document any injuries. Address any child and vulnerable adult protection issues. Carry out self-harm risk identification.
- *Medium term needs (disclosure after 7 days of assault)*—Screening for STIs at baseline and/or 2 weeks after the assault, hepatitis B vaccination as appropriate. Pregnancy testing as appropriate. Assessment of coping abilities, identify symptoms of PTSD. Practical and psychosocial support.
- *Long-term needs (disclosure after 1-year postassault)—PTSD.*

ASSESSMENT OF INJURIES

Only about 30% of sexual assault victims will have anogenital injuries. ~80% will have other bodily injuries, but most will be minor. Make sure a patient is not actively bleeding from the anogenital canal and that there is no concealed bleeding, especially if patient reports a violent assault that includes any sharp or penetrating objects. Trauma to any significant arteries in the genital tract can lead to hemorrhage which could become life-threatening. The patient must be clinically stable before transfer to a forensic service is initiated. Where the victim is not clinically stable, a forensic medical examiner or sexual offences examiner may attend the hospital to conduct the forensic examination. If injuries are minor and not actively bleeding, it is best not to clean or dress wounds until forensic samples are taken.

It is worthwhile considering tetanus booster/vaccination in contaminated wounds and antibiotic prophylaxis in human bites where the skin has been breached.

RISK OF PREGNANCY

Current method of contraception, any compliance issues, any missed/late pills, and any displacement of intrauterine contraceptive device (IUCD) following trauma. Type of sexual assault, may not be relevant in oral rape or digital penetration, recommended in either vaginal or anal rape. Last menstrual period and cycle length, previous episodes of unprotected sexual intercourse (UPSI) in that cycle, previous use of hormonal emergency contraception in the cycle, medical eligibility, drug interactions, and individual choice.

Emergency Contraception—Three Options

1. *Levonorgestrel 1.5 mg*—Progesterone only, primarily inhibits ovulation. Licensed for use within 72 hours of UPSI/contraceptive failure, can be used more than once in a cycle, regular hormonal contraception can be started immediately, relatively limited drug interactions. Give a double dose (3 mg), if BMI is >26 and weight is >70 kg; if liver enzyme-inducing drugs have been used. Advise patients to use condoms until regular contraceptive method becomes effective.
2. *Ullipristal acetate (ellaOne®) 30 mg*—Progesterone receptor modulator, inhibits or delays ovulation. Licensed for use up to 120 hours from UPSI. Avoid, if any hormonal contraceptive use in the last 7 days, in women using liver enzyme-inducing drugs, in severe asthma controlled by glucocorticoid steroids, if currently using antacids. Must wait 5 days before starting regular hormonal contraception. Advise patients to use condoms until regular contraceptive method becomes effective.
3. *Copper-bearing intrauterine device with antibiotic prophylaxis—method of choice*—Copper is toxic to the ovum and sperm, works primarily by inhibiting fertilization through changes in endometrium (aseptic inflammation). Effective immediately after insertion, can be used within the first 5 days (120 hours) following first UPSI or within 5 days from the earliest estimated date of ovulation. Can be used with severe hepatic impairment or with enzyme inducing drugs. It is important that antibiotic prophylaxis is given in the circumstances of sexual assault.

SEXUALLY TRANSMITTED INFECTIONS

Risk of transmission of chlamydia, gonorrhea, syphilis, hepatitis B and C, and HIV during sexual assault must be addressed. Screening before the earliest incubation period of these infections can yield results that may be difficult to interpret, i.e., if a positive result is due to infected semen in the genital tract, or was the patient already positive for the infection before the assault. Antibiotic prophylaxis (for gonorrhea and chlamydia) can be considered in those who requires an emergency intrauterine device fitting or is unable to attend or access screening (e.g., a patient that is likely to miss appointments, the alleged suspect is known to have an infection, or foreign travel where medical care is difficult to access). A routine screen should be organized for approximately 10–14 days after assault.

Postexposure Prophylaxis—Human Immunodeficiency Virus Postexposure Prophylaxis after Sexual Exposure

At higher risk of HIV transmission are: Suspect is known to have HIV and is not on antiretroviral therapy, suspect is from an area of high prevalence, suspect is a male known to have had sex with other men, suspect is a known intravenous drug user, breaches in mucosal barriers following trauma. PEPSE should be started as soon as possible, ideally within the first 24 hours but not beyond 72 hours of exposure, once HIV has crossed the mucosal barrier. The course lasts 28 days, consists two medications, Truvada + Raltegravir.

HEPATITIS B VACCINATION

May have a protective effect if administered within 6 weeks of the assault. An accelerated schedule with three vaccines is given within 1 month (at exposure, 1-week postexposure, and 3 weeks postexposure) is favored.

MENTAL HEALTH ASSESSMENT

An assessment of suicide risk is advised. Any mental health diagnosis, history of self-harm and suicide attempts need to be documented. Short-term psychological responses include intrusive memories, flashbacks, anxiety and fear, anger and irritability, sleep difficulties and nightmares, avoidance and withdrawal, low mood and depression, dissociation, shame and guilt, self-blame, low self-esteem, and sexual and relationship difficulties.

POST-TRAUMATIC STRESS DISORDER

People who are sexually assaulted are more likely to develop PTSD than any other trauma. The diagnostic criteria for PTSD [Diagnostic and Statistical Manual of Mental Disorders, Fourth Edition (DSM-IV)] is—Person experiences, witnesses or is confronted by an event that involves actual or threatened death or serious injury, or a threat to physical integrity of self or others and response-involved fear, helplessness, and horror, preexistent re-experiencing, persistent avoidance of stimuli associated with trauma and numbing of general responsiveness, and persistent symptoms of increased arousal. Duration >1 month, and disturbance causes clinically significant distress or impairment in social, occupational, or areas of functioning.

IMMEDIATE MANAGEMENT CHECKLIST

Be sensitive and empathetic, maintain the patient's dignity and respect their wishes, an appropriate environment for history taking and examination, assess for acute mental health concerns, assess injuries, treat serious or potentially serious injuries, offer emergency contraceptive, offer postexposure prophylaxis (PEP) for HIV, hepatitis B vaccination, consent from the patient, and refer to sexual assault center.

Forensic Considerations

Confidentiality and choice, consent to treatment and collection of specimens, collection of forensic specimens, collection of evidence, and medical care.

Forensic Samples

Oral—within 48 hours (2 days), vaginal—in 168 hours (7 days), anal—within 72 hours (3 days), digital penetration of any orifice—within 12-48 hours, skin swabs—within 48 hours (2 days) or up to 168 hours (7 days) if not washed. *For toxicology (drugs and alcohol):* Urine should be taken if incident occurred within 5 days (120 hours) or, if it is a suspected drug-facilitated sexual assault, for up to 14 days from alleged assault, blood should be taken within 3 days (72 hours). Hair sample for toxicology—in 6 months.

Absence of Injuries

May be due to no injuries sustained as a result of the alleged assault, any injury healed in the time elapsed from the alleged assault to the examination, injuries not yet appeared (for instance, bruising can take up to 48 hours to develop) or false allegation.

SUGGESTED READING

1. BASHH. Guidelines. Available from https://www.bashh.org/resources/guidelines.
2. Long L, Butler B. Sexual assault. Obstet Gynaecol. 2018;20: 87-93.

CHAPTER 49

Bacterial Vaginosis

BACTERIAL VAGINOSIS

The most common cause of abnormal vaginal discharge in reproductive age women. Prevalence 5–50%, 12–15% in pregnant women.

ETIOLOGY

Normally, the vaginal pH is <4.5, but here it becomes >4.5 (reaches ~6). Also, the predominant bacteria in healthy vagina, i.e., *Lactobacilli* becomes over dominated by many anaerobic and facultative anaerobic bacteria, with concentrations up to thousand-fold greater—*Gardnerella vaginalis*, *Prevotella* spp., *Mycoplasma hominis*, and *Mobiluncus* spp.

RISK FACTORS

Vaginal douching, black race, recent change of sex partner, and smoking. Presence of sexually transmitted infection (STI), e.g., chlamydia or herpes.

CLINICAL FEATURES: SYMPTOMS

- Offensive fishy smelling vaginal discharge
- Not associated with soreness, itching, or irritation
- Many women (approximately 50%) are asymptomatic

SIGNS

Thin, white, homogeneous discharge, coating the walls of the vagina and vestibule. Usually not associated with signs of inflammation.

COMPLICATIONS

*Bacterial vaginosis (BV) is **not** sexually transmitted but there are associations between BV, STIs, and other genital infections.* ↑association with pelvic inflammatory disease (PID) (∴ routine STI screening should be offered), human immunodeficiency virus (HIV), postmedical termination of pregnancy (MTP) endometritis, posthysterectomy vault cuff cellulitis and abscess but its treatment in asymptomatic patients does not ↓ risks. In pregnancy, it is association with late miscarriage, preterm birth, preterm premature rupture of membranes, and postpartum endometritis.

DIAGNOSIS

Amsel Criteria

Three out of four criteria should be present:

1. Thin, white, homogeneous discharge
2. Clue cells on microscopy of wet mount
3. pH of vaginal fluid >4.5
4. Fishy odor on adding alkali (10% KOH)

Hay/Ison (*Grade 1–3*) Criteria (BASHH) or Nugent Score (*Grade 0–4, Gold Standard*)

Evaluated by Gram-stained vaginal smear:

- *Grade 1 (normal): Lactobacillus* morphotypes predominate
- *Grade 2 (intermediate):* Mixed flora with some *Lactobacilli* present, but *Gardnerella* or *Mobiluncus* morphotypes also present
- *Grade 3 (BV):* Predominantly *Gardnerella* and/or *Mobiluncus*, few/absent *Lactobacilli*.
- *Grade 0:* No bacteria present.
- *Grade 4:* Gram-positive cocci predominate.

MANAGEMENT

General advice—Avoid vaginal douching, shampoo, shower gel, or antiseptics.

Treatment recommended for symptomatic/those undergoing surgical procedures:

- Metronidazole 400 mg twice daily for 5–7 days (A) or
- Metronidazole 2 g single oral dose (A) or
- Intravaginal Metronidazole gel (0.75%) once daily for 5 days (A) or

- Intravaginal Clindamycin cream (2%) once daily for 7 days (A).
- *Alternative treatment:*
  - Clindamycin 300 mg twice daily for 7 days (A) or
  - Tinidazole 2 g single dose (A).

PRECAUTION

Avoid alcohol with both oral and topical Metronidazole during treatment as well as 1 week after treatment completion due to Disulfiram-like reaction. Clindamycin cream can weaken condoms during treatment and pseudomembranous colitis is reported with both oral and Clindamycin cream.

No evidence of teratogenicity from Metronidazole during the first trimester of pregnancy (Ia).

FOLLOW-UP

A test of cure is not required if symptoms resolve.

SUGGESTED READING

1. BASHH Guidelines. (2012). Bacterial Vaginosis. Available from https://www.bashh.org/resources/guidelines.

CHAPTER 50

Vulvovaginal Candidiasis

Most common causative agent—*Candida albicans* (80–90%).

Acute vulvovaginal candidiasis (VVC): First or single isolated presentation of VVC signs and symptoms of acute vulvovaginitis and *Candida* spp. detected by microscopy and/or culture.

Recurrent VVC: At least ≥4 symptomatic episodes/12 months with two episodes confirmed by microscopy or culture (at least one positive culture with moderate or heavy growth of *Candida* spp.).

RISK FACTORS

- Poorly-controlled diabetes mellitus
- Immunosuppression
- Endogenous and exogenous estrogen [including pregnancy, hormone replacement therapy (HRT) and possibly the combined oral contraceptive pill]
- Recent antibiotic use causing a disturbance in the vaginal flora.

CLINICAL FEATURES

- Symptoms:
  - Vulval itch
  - Nonoffensive vaginal discharge
  - Soreness or burning
  - Superficial dyspareunia
- Signs:
  - Erythema
  - Fissuring
  - Swelling/edema
  - Vaginal discharge, typically nonoffensive and curdy but may be thin or absent
  - May be associated with satellite lesions and excoriation marks.

DIAGNOSIS

By clinical features supported by laboratory confirmation from a vaginal sample.

DIFFERENTIAL DIAGNOSIS

Lichen sclerosus, vulvo-/vestibulodynia, contact dermatitis/eczema, and chronic lichen simplex/chronic eczema.

Clinical examination of external genitalia to exclude alternative or coexisting vulvovaginal pathologies and syndromic management should be done. If clinical examination is not possible it requires self-collected vaginal swab for *microscopy* and/or *culture* is a reasonable alternative. Empirical treatment for acute VVC based on the reported symptoms may be given. Screening for sexually transmitted infection (STI) in the presence of risk factors.

MANAGEMENT

General—careful review of their daily routine hygiene (washing hair in bath water or excessive cleaning, wearing incorrectly fitted clothing made from nonbreathable fabric, using intermenstrual or daily panty liners, and vaginal douching); *avoid use* of local irritants such as perfumed soaps or wipes, *use* an emollient for personal hygiene as a soap substitute, a moisturizer and a barrier cream; avoid sex until symptoms have improved particularly if there is fissuring of the skin.

In recurrent VVC, screen for the following:

- Diabetes with urinalysis, random blood glucose, or HbA1c (Grade 2C)
- Iron-deficiency anemia with a full blood count or serum ferritin (Grade 2C)

TREATMENT

Acute Vulvovaginal Candidiasis

Recommended regimen: Fluconazole 150 mg as a single dose, orally (1B).

Recommended topical regimen (if oral therapy contra-indicated): Clotrimazole pessary 500 mg as a single dose, intravaginally (1B).

Alternative regimens: Clotrimazole pessary 200 mg intravaginally at night for three consecutive nights (1C).

Treatment considerations: Oral therapies must be avoided in pregnancy, risk of pregnancy, and breastfeeding. Intravaginal and topical treatments can also damage latex condoms and diaphragms with risk of unwanted pregnancy. A medication history should be taken to rule out that oral Fluconazole and other azoles can interact with other medications (Cisapride, Astemizole, Pimozide, Quinidine, and Erythromycin—all prolong the QT interval). Since Fluconazole is associated with prolongation of the QT interval on the electrocardiogram, risk assessment should be done before prescribing two or more drugs associated with QT prolongation [increasing age, female sex, cardiac disease, and some metabolic disturbances (notably hypokalemia) predispose to QT prolongation].

Recurrent VVC: Recommended regimen—

- *Induction:* Fluconazole 150 mg orally every 72 hourly, three doses (1A)
- *Maintenance:* Fluconazole 150 mg orally once a week for 6 months (1A)

Nonalbicans Candida species and azole resistance: Recommended regimen—Nystatin pessaries 100,000 units intravaginally at night for 12–14 consecutive nights (1B).

Overall cure rate—80–90%.

FOLLOW-UP

- Follow-up and test of cure for patients with acute VVC is unnecessary if symptoms resolve.
- Recurrent VVC should be advised to return if they experience poor or partial response to therapy; repeat microscopy and culture is indicated to assess for microbiological cure or new resistance.
- Patients who demonstrate microbiological response but not clinical response to therapy should be reassessed for alternative causes of their symptoms.

CONTACT TRACING AND TREATMENT

No evidence to support treatment of asymptomatic male sexual partners in acute or recurrent VVC.

SUGGESTED READING

1. BASHH Guideline. (2019). Management of vulvovaginal candidiasis. [online] Available from https://www.bashh.org/resources/22/vulvovaginal_candidiasis_2019/ [Last accessed September, 2024].

CHAPTER 51

Trichomonas Vaginalis

Flagellated protozoan, exclusively transmitted through sexual intercourse.

CLINICAL FEATURES

Symptoms

- ~50% are asymptomatic.
- Vaginal discharge, vulval itching, dysuria, or offensive odor.
- Lower abdominal discomfort or vulval ulceration.

Signs

- Vaginal discharge (70%), consistency varies from thin and scanty to profuse and thick.
- Classical frothy yellow discharge occurs in 10–30% of women.
- Vulvitis and vaginitis, ~15% may have normal appearance.
- ~2% of patients have strawberry cervix appearance.

COMPLICATIONS

During pregnancy ↑risk of preterm labor, low birth weight (LBW), puerperal sepsis; but screening of asymptomatic individuals for *Trichomonas vaginalis* (TV) infection in pregnancy is **not** recommended (Grade 1B).

DIAGNOSIS

Testing for TV done if case of vaginal discharge or e/o vulvovaginitis (Grade 1A), by microscopy/nucleic acid amplification test (NAAT)/culture.

In symptomatic patients, a swab taken from the posterior fornix of the vagina at the time of speculum examination (and mixed with a small drop of saline on a glass slide with coverslip placed on top, this wet preparation read within 10 minutes of collection, as the trichomonads will quickly lose motility and difficult to identify) is recommended (Grade 1A).

Self-administered vaginal swabs give similar results to clinician-taken swabs using NAATs and is the test of choice if microscopy not being performed (Grade 1A).

MANAGEMENT

General: Sexual partner should be treated simultaneously (Grade 1B). Patients should be advised to avoid unprotected sexual intercourse for at least 1 week, until they and their partner have completed treatment and follow-up.

Screen for other sexually transmitted infections (STIs) (Grade 1A).

TREATMENT

Recommended Regimen (Grade 1A)

Metronidazole 400 mg twice daily for 7 days. Alcohol should be avoided during treatment and till 48 hours postlast dose, as it may cause Disulfiram-like reaction.

Alternative regimens—Metronidazole 2 g orally in a single dose (Grade 2A).

Pregnancy and breastfeeding—400 mg oral Metronidazole twice daily for 7 days in preference to the use of short high-dose regimens which are not recommended during pregnancy (Grade 1A).

In cases of treatment failure, check for—Compliance and exclude vomiting of Metronidazole. Sexual history for possibility of reinfection and ensure if partner(s) have been treated.

Treatment protocol for nonresponse to standard TV therapy:

- Repeat course of 7-day standard therapy.
- Higher dose course of Nitroimidazole (Grade 2B)
- Very high dose course of Nitroimidazole and very high dose course of Nitroimidazole with intravaginal Nitroimidazole or Paromomycin cream (Grade 2D).

Secnidazole is a second-generation 5-Nitroimidazole product with a broad spectrum of activity against anaerobic bacteria and longer half-life than Metronidazole, making it suitable for single-dose therapy.

FOLLOW-UP

Tests of cure only recommended if patient remains symptomatic following treatment, or if symptoms recur (Grade 2C). Optimum timing of NAAT for *Trichomonas vaginalis* test of cure is 4 weeks after the start of treatment.

MANAGEMENT OF SEXUAL PARTNERS

Contact tracing and partner notification—Current partners and any sexual partner(s) in last 4 weeks should be offered treatment, as well as full STI screening and human immunodeficiency virus (HIV) testing.

SUGGESTED READING

1. BASHH Guideline. (2021). Management of *Trichomonas vaginalis.* [online] Available from https://www.bashh.org/resources/20/trichomonas_vaginalis_2021/ [Last accessed September, 2024].

CHAPTER 52

Gonorrhea

ETIOLOGY

Gram-negative diplococcus *Neisseria gonorrhoeae* (NG). Sites of infection—columnar epithelium lined mucous membranes of urethra, endocervix, rectum, pharynx, and conjunctiva. Highly transmissible infection can lead to serious sequelae if untreated, even in asymptomatic patients.

TRANSMISSION

Direct inoculation of infected secretions from one mucous membrane to other.

CLINICAL FEATURES

Symptoms

Dysuria (without frequency), vaginal discharge, pain lower abdomen, intermenstrual bleeding and menorrhagia; anal discharge, and perianal/anal pain/discomfort.

Signs

Mucopurulent endocervical discharge, and easily induced endocervical bleeding.

COMPLICATIONS

Pelvic inflammatory diseases (PID), skin lesions, arthralgia, arthritis, and tenosynovitis (disseminated gonococcal infection). Uncomplicated limited to urogenital tract, anorectum, and oropharynx.

DIAGNOSIS

Detection of NG by nucleic acid amplification tests (NAATs more sensitive > culture) or by culture. Microscopy of Gram-stained genital specimens for direct visualization of NG as Gram-negative diplococci within polymorphonuclear leukocytes (**not** recommended due to low sensitivity).

Recommended optimal specimen is self-collected or clinician-collected vulvovaginal swabs (better than endocervical swabs) (Grade 1A).

Pharyngeal sampling if genital infection confirms Ceftriaxone resistant strain (Grade 1D).

Individuals diagnosed NG by NAAT should have cultures taken for antimicrobial susceptibility testing prior to treatment, due to ↑antimicrobial resistance (Grade 1D).

TIMING OF TESTING

Individuals presenting within 2 weeks of sexual contact with an infected partner should return for repeat testing after this *window period* if epidemiological treatment not given (Grade 1D).

Screen for other sexually transmitted infections (STIs)—chlamydia (40% coinfection, ∴ presumptive treatment of chlamydia should be given at same time), human immunodeficiency virus (HIV), and syphilis.

MANAGEMENT

General

Counseling regarding health implications for patient and their sexual partner, and they should avoid sexual intercourse till >7 days of treatment completion (Grade1D).

Recommended treatment of uncomplicated anogenital and pharyngeal infection:

- *When antimicrobial susceptibility is not known prior to treatment:* Ceftriaxone 1 g intramuscularly as a single dose (Grade 1C).
- *When antimicrobial susceptibility is known prior to treatment:* Ciprofloxacin 500 mg orally as a single dose (Grade 1A).

Alternative treatment: Cefixime 400 mg orally single dose + Azithromycin 2 g orally (Grade 1B), only advisable if intra-muscular (IM) injection is contraindicated or refused or allergic to it.

Treatment of complicated infections—Gonococcal PID: Ceftriaxone 1 g IM as a single dose in addition to the regimen chosen to treat PID.

Disseminated Gonococcal Infection

Ceftriaxone 1 g IM or intravenous (IV) every 24 hours, or Cefotaxime 1 g IV every 8 hours.

This can be switched 24–48 hours after symptoms improvement to one of the following oral regimens for 7 days:

- Cefixime 400 mg twice daily
- Ciprofloxacin 500 mg twice daily
- Ofloxacin 400 mg twice daily

Pregnancy and Breastfeeding

- Ceftriaxone 1 g IM as a single dose (Grade 1A)
- Spectinomycin 2 g IM as a single dose (Grade 1A)
- Azithromycin 2 g as a single oral dose (Grade 1B).

Treatment of sexual partners—All partners within last 3 months should be notified and treated according to their time of presentation. If they present >14 days of exposure, treat only if positive for NG.

If presenting within 14 days of exposure, epidemiological treatment based on clinical risk assessment. If asymptomatic, no epidemiological treatment, repeat testing 2 weeks after exposure and treat if positive.

FOLLOW-UP AND TEST OF CURE

All patients diagnosed with gonorrhea should be advised to return for test of cure (TOC) if they have:

- Persistent symptoms or signs
- Pharyngeal infection
- Treated with other than first-line recommended regimen (antimicrobial susceptibility unknown)
- Acquired infection in Asia-Pacific region (antimicrobial susceptibility unknown)

A positive TOC could be due to treatment failure, reinfection, or residual nonviable organism and it should be interpreted in the clinical context.

SUGGESTED READING

1. BASHH Guideline. (2018). Gonorrhoea. [online] Available from https://www.bashh.org/resources/14/gonorrhoea_2018/ [Last accessed September, 2024].

CHAPTER 53

Chlamydia

ETIOLOGY

Obligate intracellular bacterium *Chlamydia trachomatis* (CT). Most commonly reported, curable bacterial sexually transmitted infections (STI). Infection primarily through penetrative sexual intercourse, although it can be detected in the conjunctiva and nasopharynx without concomitant genital infection. If untreated, infection may persist or resolve spontaneously (~50% in 12 months).

CLINICAL FEATURES

Symptoms

- In majority, infection is asymptomatic
- Increased vaginal discharge
- Postcoital and intermenstrual bleeding
- Dysuria
- Lower abdominal pain
- Deep dyspareunia

Signs

- Mucopurulent cervicitis with or without contact bleeding
- Pelvic tenderness
- Cervical motion tenderness

Extragenital infection—anal discharge and anorectal discomfort, conjunctival low-grade irritation, and pharyngeal usually asymptomatic.

DIAGNOSIS

Although no test is 100% sensitive or specific, nucleic acid amplification test (NAATs) are more sensitive, and specific than enzyme immunoassays (EIAs). Vulvovaginal swabs is the specimen of choice in women (Level IIa, Grade B). Endocervical swabs are less sensitive than vulvovaginal swab and require speculum examination.

First catch urine is less sensitive than vulvovaginal/endocervical swabs.

Extragenital sampling: Rectal swabs and pharyngeal swabs—NAATs are the choice for both genital and extragenital samples, though the sensitivities are variable (Level IIa, Grade B).

Also screen for other STIs—human immunodeficiency virus (HIV), gonorrhea, and syphilis. *Mycoplasma genitalium* is emerging as a significant sexually transmitted pathogen and coinfection rates of 3–15% with chlamydia have been reported.

COMPLICATIONS

- Pelvic inflammatory disease (PID), endometritis, and salpingitis
- Tubal infertility
- Ectopic pregnancy
- Sexually acquired reactive arthritis (SARA) (<1%)
- Perihepatitis

MANAGEMENT

Goal of treatment to prevent complications, ↓risk of transmission to others, resolve symptoms, and prevent reinfection.

Recommended Regimen

Uncomplicated urogenital infection (Level Ia, Grade A) and pharyngeal infection (Level IV, Grade C):

- Doxycycline 100 mg BD for 7 days (contraindicated in pregnancy) or
- Azithromycin 1 g orally as a single dose, followed by 500 mg once daily for 2 days.

Alternative Treatment

Ofloxacin 200 mg BD or 400 mg OD for 7 days (Level Ib, Grade A) or Erythromycin 500 mg BD for 10–14 days (Level IV, Grade C).

PREGNANCY AND BREASTFEEDING

Doxycycline and Ofloxacin are contraindicated in pregnancy.

Recommended regimens (Level Ia, Grade A):

- Azithromycin 1 g orally as a single dose, followed by 500 mg once daily for 2 days

- Erythromycin 500 mg four times daily for 7 days
- Amoxicillin 500 mg three times a day for 7 days

FOLLOW-UP AND TEST OF CURE

Not routinely recommended for uncomplicated genital chlamydia infection, because residual, nonviable chlamydial deoxyribonucleic acid (DNA) may be detected by NAAT for 3–5 weeks following treatment. Refrain from sexual activity till 7-day after treatment completed, symptoms resolved and sexual partners treated.

Test of cure is recommended at 4 weeks after treatment in pregnancy, where poor compliance is suspected and where symptoms persist.

All treated should undergo retesting >3 months to identify reinfection.

CONTACT TRACING AND TREATMENT

All sexual partners treatment, within last 2–3 months should be notified and offered, full STI screening, including HIV testing and if indicated, hepatitis B screening and vaccination (Level IV, Grade C).

SUGGESTED READING

1. BASHH Guideline. Chlamydia. [online] Available from https://www.bashh.org/resources/15/chlamydia_2015.

NOTES

SECTION 11

Contraception

Section Authors: *Mridu Sinha, Babita Kumari, Sunaina Chandra*

CHAPTER 54

Emergency Contraception

DEFINITION

A method of contraception used as an emergency procedure to prevent pregnancy before menstruation is missed, following unprotected sexual intercourse (UPSI) or expected failure of contraception. Also called "postcoital" contraception/"morning-after" pill. Not a regular contraception due to high failure-rate/high incidence of irregular bleeding.

INDICATIONS

- Aged couple who meets infrequently.
- Single act of sexual exposure in young girls.
- Pregnancy apprehended due to ruptured condom, detection of defect in diaphragm after use or premature ejaculation in coitus interruptus.
- Rape/incest
- Unprotected isolated intercourse occurs in couples using conventional methods.

MECHANISM

Stops or postpones ovulation, interferes with implantation, and decreases longevity of blastocyst.

Agents which do not interfere with fertilization but act on blastocyst before or soon after implantation → *interceptives*. Those which interfere with early gestation before or soon after missing periods → contragestives.

METHODS

- Hormonal—Levonorgestrel (LNG) only pills, Ulipristal acetate (UPA) (Fibristal), combined (OGN + PGN) pills ("Yuzpe" regime).
- Mechanical—Copper T (Cu T) intrauterine device (IUCD).

RECOMMENDATIONS

Cu-IUCD—Most effective method of emergency contraception (EC), only method that is effective after ovulation. It should be inserted within 5 days after UPSI in a cycle, or within 5 days of earliest estimated date of ovulation, whichever is later. Also, an effective ongoing contraception and not known to be affected by body mass index (BMI)/weight or by other drugs.

Oral EC—Offered as soon as possible (ASAP) after UPSI if a Cu-IUD is not appropriate or is not acceptable. It is unlikely to be effective if taken >120 hours after the last UPSI, as viable sperm are present in the upper genital tract for only about 5 days after UPSI. It acts by delaying ovulation, i.e., oral EC is not effective after ovulation has taken place.

Factors to be considered for oral EC—Overall UPA-EC is more effective >LNG-EC, but effectiveness of UPA-EC can be reduced if a woman has recently taken a progestogen or planning to start hormonal contraception (LNG-EC favored). LNG-EC less effective if BMI >26 kg/m^2 or weight >70 kg, either UPA-EC or a double dose (3 mg) of LNG-EC is recommended. Both UPA-EC and LNG-EC can be used more than once in the same cycle. Quick start of suitable contraception (immediately after LNG-EC or >5 days after UPA-EC) should be offered and follow-up pregnancy testing arranged. All requesting EC should be assessed as to their risk of sexually transmitted infection (STI).

OPTIONS

- *Mechanical—Cu T 380A, ML Cu250, and ML Cu 375 IUCD*—inserted postcoitally up to 5 days after exposure. Mode of action—biochemical and histological changes in endometrium, toxic to the ovum and sperm, damages blastocyst directly at time of implantation. Advantages—can continue as method of ongoing contraception, can be used if estrogen contraindicated, and effective immediately after insertion. Used within the first 5 days (120 hours) following first UPSI or within 5 days from the earliest estimated date of ovulation, can be used with severe hepatic impairment, or with enzyme inducing drugs. It is important that antibiotic prophylaxis is given in sexual assault. Disadvantages—Bleeding, pain, expulsion, perforation, and pelvic inflammatory disease (PID)/sexually transmitted disease (STD)/human immunodeficiency disease (HIV). Failure rate—1:1,000.

- *Levonorgestrel 1.5 mg*—"Pill 72" "Unwanted" "emergency contraceptive pill", progesterone only, primarily inhibits ovulation, licensed for use within 72 hours of UPSI/contraceptive failure, can be used more than once in a cycle, regular hormonal contraception can be started immediately, and relatively limited drug interactions. *Give a double dose (3 mg):* If BMI is >26 kg/m^2, weight is >70 kg; if liver enzyme-inducing drugs have been used. *Avoid:* For 5 days if UPA has already been taken. Advise patients to use condoms until regular contraceptive method becomes effective. Failure rate—1-3%.
- *Ullipristal acetate (ellaOne) 30 mg*—Progesterone receptor modulator, inhibits or delays ovulation, licensed for use up to 120 hours from UPSI. *Avoid:* If any hormonal contraceptive use in the last 7 days, if using liver enzyme-inducing drugs, in severe asthma controlled by glucocorticoid steroids, and if currently using medication that increases gastric pH. Must wait 5 days before starting regular hormonal contraception. Advise patients to use condoms until regular contraceptive method becomes effective. Failure rate—1-2%.
- *Combined OGN + PGN pill [not recommended by faculty of sexual and reproductive health (FSRH)]*— Two types:
  1. High dose—Ethinylestradiol (EE) (50 µg) + LNG (250 µg)/dL-norgestrel (500 µg)—two pills followed by other two pills after 12 hours.
  2. Low dose—EE (30 µg) + LNG (150 µg)/dL-norgestrel (300 µg)—four pills followed by four more pills after 12 hours.

  Mode of action—inhibition/delay of ovulation, prevention of implantation in altered endometrium. Risks—vaginal adenosis/adenocarcinoma, limb defect/CVS defect in children. Side effects—nausea, vomiting, irregular bleeding per vaginum, headache, dizziness, breast tenderness, and fatigue.

SUGGESTED READING

1. FSRH Guideline. (2017). Emergency contraception. [online] Available from https://www.fsrh.org/Public/Public/Standards-and-Guidance/fsrh-guidelines-and-statements.aspx?hkey=641ed042-35d8-48c0-96ee-968f5e449241.

CHAPTER 55

Long-acting Reversible Contraceptives

DEFINITION

Those contraceptive methods that require administration less than once in a month/a menstrual cycle, e.g., copper intrauterine device (IUD), Mirena, injection Depot Medroxyprogesterone Acetate (DMPA), and implants.

More cost-effective as compared to pills, and daily compliance not required.

INTRAUTERINE CONTRACEPTIVE DEVICE

Table 1 shows comparison between copper intrauterine contraceptive device (IUCD) and hormonal IUCD, i.e., Mirena.

CLINICAL ASSESSMENT

History Taking

Menstrual history, contraception history, sexual history, obstetric history, medical history, surgical history, and family history. Exclude pregnancy, do sexually transmitted infection (STI) risk assessment. Inform—contraceptive efficacy, duration of use, procedure of initiation and discontinuation, noncontraceptive benefits, risks and side-effects, and when to seek medical help.

Treatment of abnormal uterine bleeding (AUB-I)—Nonsteroidal Anti-Inflammatory Drugs (NSAIDs) if due

TABLE 1: Intrauterine contraception.

Features	*Cu-T 380A/ML-375 S*	*LNG-IUS (Mirena)*
Mode of action	Copper causes endometrial inflammatory reaction, i.e., hostile for implantation, also toxic to sperm and ovum, and reduced rates of blastocyst formation. Altered copper content of cervical mucus inhibit sperm penetration	LNG interferes with implantation, reduced rates of blastocyst formation and makes cervical mucus thick for sperm penetration, changes in intercellular junctions between the endometrial epithelial and stromal cells, and an increase in endometrial phagocytic cells
Life-term	5/10 years	5 years (Jaydess—3 years)
Failure rate	<2%	<1%
Other uses (noncontraceptive benefits)	Emergency contraception	HMB, HRT (with estrogen patch), dysmenorrhea, adenomyosis, and endometriosis
Releases	Copper ions are released locally inside uterus, no systemic absorption	52 mg LNG-IUS (Mirena) releases (approximate) 20 µg LNG/day—5 years [13.5 mg LNG-IUS (Jaydess) releases 14 µg/day—3 years]
Insertion method ("no-touch technology") and effective	• "Withdrawal method"—copper T (Cu-T) • "Push method"—Multiload • Postpartum—Kelly forceps • Immediately after insertion	Bayer inserter—Load by pushing slider to front—set flange—insert till flange 1.5–2 cm from cervix (Cx)—release arms by pushing slider down—advance to fundus—takes 1 week to be effective
Side-effects	AUB (irregular, prolonged, and frequent bleeding), pain, and infection	Breast tenderness/pain, headache, acne, and AUB (~to Cu-T, infrequent bleeding, and amenorrhea at 1 year)

(AUB: abnormal uterine bleeding; HMB: heavy menstrual bleeding; HRT: hormone replacement therapy; LNG-IUS: Levonorgestrel-releasing intrauterine system)

to copper T (Cu-T), and combined oral contraceptive pill (COCP) for 3 months if intrauterine system (IUS).

Cu-T with *pelvic inflammatory disease* (PID) → no routine removal, except if not responding to treatment after 72 hours of antibiotics [with additional emergency contraception (EC) if unprotected sexual intercourse (UPSI) in last 7 days].

Insertion timings [check World Health Organization (WHO) eligibility criteria to rule out contraindications—active PID, sexually transmitted disease (STD), genital tuberculosis (TB), undiagnosed AUB, and distorted cavity), and valid consent].

- Postplacental—within 10 minutes of placental delivery
- Postpartum—within 48 hours of delivery
- Postabortal—immediately after surgical method/expulsion in medical method
- Interval—within 4–7 days of menses
- Emergency—up to 5 days postovulation

Follow-up after first menses postinsertion, or signs of infection, pain, bleeding, late menses, and nonpalpable (missing) threads/feeling the stem.

Complications—ectopic, perforation (2/1,000), expulsion (1/20), and ovarian cysts (Mirena).

For women with cardiac disease, involve a cardiologist, and should be fitted in a hospital setting if a vasovagal reaction occur especially high-risk women with single ventricle circulation, Eisenmenger physiology, tachycardia, or preexisting bradycardia.

PROGESTOGEN-ONLY INJECTABLES (INJECTION DEPOT MEDROXYPROGESTERONE ACETATE/ NORETHISTERONE ENANTHATE)

DMPA (1) Depo-Provera [150 mg Medroxyprogesterone Acetate (MPA)/1 mL] deep intramuscular (IM), (2) Sayana Press (104 mg MPA in 0.65 mL) subcutaneous (SC), injection, (3) Norethisterone Enanthate (NET-EN) Noristerat (200 mg in 1 mL) IM injection.

Mode of action—inhibiting ovulation, effect on cervical mucus limiting sperm penetration, and changes to the endometrium make it an unfavorable environment for implantation.

Timing of injection—D1-5 of menses, <D-5 of first/second trimester miscarriage, and >D-21 of delivery. Repeat dose of IM DMPA, SC DMPA, and NET-EN at 12 weeks, 13 weeks, and 8 weeks, respectively. Faculty of sexual and reproductive healthcare (FSRH)—Women should be advised to return every 13 weeks for a repeat injection of IM or SC DMPA, and it can be administered up to 7 days late (up to 14 weeks after the last injection) without the need for additional contraceptive precautions.

Failure rate—0.2% (2/1,000)

Noncontraceptive benefits—reduces menstrual bleeding, may cause amenorrhea in heavy menstrual bleeding (HMB), reduces pain (dysmenorrhea, endometriosis), and reduce the severity of sickle crisis pain.

Side-effects—altered bleeding patterns (amenorrhea, infrequent bleeding, spotting, and prolonged bleeding), small loss of bone mineral density (BMD) (reversible after discontinuation), weight gain [<18 years of age with body mass index (BMI) ≥30 kg/m^2], delayed return of fertility, acne, decreased libido, mood swings, headache, and hot flushes and vaginitis have been reported with use of DMPA. Injection site reactions appear to be more common with use of SC DMPA than with use of IM DMPA.

Management of problematic/unscheduled bleeding: After ruling out other causes (STI, cervical smear, etc.). Combined oral contraceptive pill (COC) for 3 months (cyclical/continuous) or tablet Mefenamic acid 500 mg TDS for 5 days.

NB. For women taking antiepileptic or antiretroviral drugs that induce liver enzymes DMPA may be an appropriate method of contraception because its efficacy is unaffected.

PROGESTOGEN-ONLY-IMPLANTS

Etonogestrel-implant (ENG-IMP) (Implanon, Nexplanon) is a single-rod subdermal contraceptive implant that releases the progestogen ENG, licensed for 3 years of use for contraception. Two-rod [each contains 75 mg Levonorgestrel (LNG)] implant *Jadelle;* six-rod (each with 36 mg LNG) *Norplant* work for 5 years (release rate 30–40 μg/day).

Single, flexible, nonbiodegradable, radio-opaque plastic rod, supplied preloaded in a sterile, single-use insertion device, core contains 68 mg ENG (the active metabolite of Desogestrel, a 19-Nortestosterone derivative), and Barium sulfate for radio-opacity. ENG release rate varies from 60 to 70 μg/day in weeks 5–6 to 35–45 μg/day at the end of the first year, and 25–30 μg/day at the end of the 3rd year.

Mode of action—It acts by suppressing ovulation, makes endometrium thin, inactive or weakly proliferative, and cervical mucus hostile for sperm penetration. The contraceptive effect is lost rapidly after removal.

Timing of insertion—D1–5 of a natural menstrual cycle, by D-5 postabortion or by D-21 postpartum (without need for additional contraceptive precaution).

Procedure—Insertion must be subdermal. With the individual lying on their back with the arm (usually the nondominant arm) abducted to 90°, the elbow flexed and the hand behind the head, the point of insertion is identified by measuring 8–10 cm proximally from the medial epicondyle along the sulcal line and then 3–5 cm posteriorly from that point over triceps, and perpendicular to the sulcal line. The inserter is advanced proximally from this insertion point, parallel to the sulcal line, and in the subdermal layer.

Failure rate—0.05% (5/10,000)

Noncontraceptive benefits—improves dysmenorrhea and endometriosis-associated pain.

Contraceptive efficacy of ENG-IMP could be reduced during use of the enzyme-inducer, and for 28 days after stopping the enzyme-inducer.

Side-effects—Irregular, unpredictable bleeding, headache, acne, mastalgia, abdomen pain, nausea, dizziness, nervousness, and local migration (possibly small increase in risk of breast cancer). Possible complications of insertion-removal procedures include local reaction, nerve damage, deep or intramuscular insertion, and rarely, distant intravascular migration. To manage problematic bleeding, a 3-month trial of additional COC or a 5-day course of Mefenamic acid can be considered for medically eligible individuals.

Contraindications—Breast cancer, arterial thromboembolism, decompensated cirrhosis, hepatocellular tumors, and unexplained vaginal bleeding.

SUGGESTED READING

1. FSRH guidelines
2. NICE guidelines

CHAPTER 56

Unscheduled Bleeding with Hormonal Contraception

INTRODUCTION

Clinically important bleeding patterns in women aged 15–44 years.

***Scheduled** bleeding*—Menstruation or regular withdrawal bleeding with combined hormonal contraception (HC).

***Unscheduled** bleeding:*

- Frequent bleeding—>5 bleeding episodes in 90 days.
- Prolonged bleeding—≥1 bleeding episodes lasting ≥14 days.
- Irregular bleeding—between 3 and 5 episodes with <3 bleeding-free intervals of ≥14 days.
- Spotting—may not require the use of sanitary protection.
- Breakthrough bleeding (BTB)—unscheduled bleeding in women using HC.

The exact mechanism of BTB is not known, but superficial blood vessel fragility within the endometrium is a common cause. In addition, local changes in endometrial steroid response, structural integrity, tissue perfusion, and local angiogenic factors are likely to contribute.

Bleeding patterns in the first 3 months of contraception use:

- Combined hormonal contraceptives (CHC) (pill/patch/ring)—20% have irregular bleeding
- Progestogen-only pill (POP)—one-third have a change in bleeding and 1 in 10 have frequent bleeding
- Depot Medroxyprogesterone Acetate (DMPA)/Norethisterone Enanthate (NET-N)/implant—spotting, light, heavy, or prolonged bleeding are common. 35% are amenorrheic at 3 months.
- Levonorgestrel-releasing intrauterine system (LNG-IUS)—irregular, light, or heavy bleeding is common in first 6 months.

PREMETHOD COUNSELING

Before starting HC, women should be advised about the expected bleeding patterns both initially and in the longer term. If bleeding patterns are outside the expected normal patterns associated with different contraceptive methods then examination, investigation, or treatment may be indicated.

INITIAL MANAGEMENT

- A clinical history should be taken from women using HC with unscheduled bleeding to identify the possibility of an underlying cause. Current method of contraception and the duration of use, any medications that may interact with the contraceptive method, or any illness that may affect the absorption of orally administered hormones, cervical screening history, sexually transmitted infection (STI), bleeding pattern before starting HC, symptoms suggestive of an underlying cause (e.g., abdominal or pelvic pain, postcoital bleeding, dyspareunia, and heavy bleeding), and possibility of pregnancy.
- Hormonal contraceptive users with unscheduled bleeding who are at risk of STI should be tested for *Chlamydia trachomatis* and *Neisseria gonorrhoeae.*
- Cervical screening should be done with Pap smear or liquid-based cytology (LBC).
- Urine pregnancy test (UPT) if clinical history suggests the possibility of incorrect method use, drug interactions or illness, which may lead to malabsorption of oral hormones and its failure.

EXAMINATION AND INVESTIGATION

- Speculum examination should be done for women using HC with unscheduled bleeding if they have: Persistent bleeding or a change in bleeding after at least 3 months use of a method; or failed medical treatment; or if they have not undergone cervical screening. Bimanual examination should also be performed for women using HC with unscheduled bleeding if they have other symptoms (such as pain, dyspareunia, and heavy bleeding).

- In general, an endometrial biopsy may be considered in women aged ≥45 years (or in women aged <45 years with risk factors for endometrial cancer such as obesity, polycystic ovarian syndrome, Tamoxifen use, or unopposed estrogen therapy) who have persistent unscheduled bleeding ≥3 months after starting a method.
- The role of structural abnormalities (such as uterine polyps, fibroids, and ovarian cysts) as a cause of unscheduled bleeding is limited. If such a structural abnormality is suspected, a transvaginal ultrasound scan and/or hysteroscopy is indicated.

THERAPEUTIC MANAGEMENT OPTIONS

- It is not generally recommended to change a combined oral contraceptive pill (COC) in the first 3 months of use as bleeding disturbances often settle in this time. However, if COC with the lowest dose of Ethinyl Estradiol (EE) is used, then the dose of EE can be increased to a maximum of 35 µg to provide good cycle control.
- Bleeding is common in the initial months of progestogen-only method use and may settle without treatment. No evidence that changing the type and dose of Progestogen-only pill will improve bleeding, but this may help some individuals.
- For unscheduled bleeding with DMPA/NET-N, implant or LNG-IUS, who wish to continue with the method and are medically eligible, a COC may be used for up to 3 months (this can be in the usual cyclic manner or continuously without a pill-free interval).
- For women using a progestogen-only injectable contraceptive with unscheduled bleeding, Mefenamic acid (or Tranexamic acid) 500 mg twice/thrice daily for 5 days can reduce the length of a bleeding episode but has little effect on bleeding in the longer term.

SUGGESTED READING

1. FSRH Guideline. (2009). Management of unscheduled bleeding in women using hormonal contraception. [online] Available from https://www.rcog.org.uk/media/oj5fuf1u/unscheduledbleeding23092009.pdf.

CHAPTER 57

Missed Pill Management

COMBINED ORAL CONTRACEPTIVE (MONOPHASIC WITH ETHINYL ESTRADIOL AND ONLY 21 ACTIVE PILLS)—MISSED PILL MANAGEMENT

- ***Late starting after hormone free interval (HFI):*** ≥9 days since last pill—emergency contraception (EC) if unprotected sexual intercourse (UPSI) during/after HFI—take most recent missed pill as soon as possible (ASAP), continue remaining pills at usual time, alternative back-up for next 7 days till pill becomes effective (barrier/avoid sex), and follow-up urine pregnancy test (UPT).
- ***One missed pill (48–<72 hours of last pill in current pack):*** If missed in 1st week after HFI (started on time)—EC not required—take missed pill ASAP, continue remaining pills at usual time, no additional contraception (if consistent correct use in 1st week and last month before HFI). If missed in 2nd/3rd week with consistent correct use in 1st week, EC not required, take missed pill ASAP, continue remaining pills at usual time, and no additional contraception required.
- ***≥2 pills missed (≥72 hours since last active pill of current pack):*** If missed in 1st week with started on time—consider EC if UPSI in 1st week/HFI—take the most recent missed pill ASAP, continue remaining pills at usual time, alternative back-up for next 7 days till pill becomes effective (barrier/avoid sex), and follow-up UPT. If missed in 2nd/3rd week with consistent correct use in 1st week—EC not required—take the most recent missed pill ASAP, continue remaining pills at usual time, alternative back-up for next 7 days till pill becomes effective (barrier/avoid sex), and if two or more pills missed in 7 days prior to scheduled HFI, omit HFI, and continue next pack without any gap.
- ***If >7 consecutive pills missed:*** Consider EC—manage as new start contraception, consider immediate UPT, quick start new combined oral contraceptive (COC) pill (or other effective contraception), alternative back-up for next 7 days till pill becomes effective (barrier/avoid sex), and consider follow-up UPT.

SUGGESTED READING

1. FSRH CEU Guidance. (2021). Recommended actions after incorrect use of combined hormonal contraception (e.g. late or missed pills, ring, and patch). [online] Available from https://www.fsrh.org/Public/Public/Documents/fsrh-ceu-guidance-recommended-actions-after-incorrect-use.aspx.

NOTES

NOTES

SECTION 12

Surgical Skills and Postoperative Complications

Section Authors: *Mridu Sinha, Jyoti Baghel, Chanchal Choudhary*

CHAPTER 58

Enhanced Recovery Program in Gynecology

AIM AND OBJECTIVES

- Improves quality and experience of care in patients undergoing elective gynecology surgery.
- Decreases physical and psychological stress by decreasing physiological stress response and organ dysfunction caused by surgery.
- Facilitates more rapid recovery, decreasing length of hospital stay, and return to normal activity.
- Involves patients and their caretakers at every step from decision-to-delivery.

It has three important components—(1) Preoperative care, (2) Perioperative care, and (3) Postoperative care.

1. *Preoperative care*—includes risk assessment both medical and surgical and correction of modifiable risk factors such as anemia, diabetes, hypertension, asthma, etc., and medical disorders. It also deals with lifestyle factors such as increase body mass index (BMI), smoking, addiction as well as any long-standing medications such as hormones, contraceptive pills, blood thinners (Heparin/Warfarin/Aspirin/Clopidogrel), etc., and dose modification/substitution. Patient is also provided procedure-specific information and an informed consent taken including—benefits, risks, alternatives, anesthesia, and any other procedure that may be required if complications occur (BT /other specialities may be required like in ureteric/bowel injury). A comprehensive plan from date of admission till discharge is made.
2. *Perioperative care*—patient is advised admission on morning of surgery to decrease preoperative bed occupancy. Fluid fasting with complex carbohydrate drinks, till 2 hours prior to operation to avoid dehydration. No bowel preparation or long-acting sedative premedication to be given. Antibiotics prior to skin incision and venous thromboembolism (VTE) prophylaxis in presence of risk factors. Minimal access technique should be preferred and if required in open surgeries the abdominal incision should be kept as small as possible. No routine use of nasogastric tube/abdominal or vaginal drains/vaginal pack. Standard anesthetic protocol should be followed regarding type of anesthesia, optimum fluid management during surgery, and avoidance of intraoperative hypothermia. Also standardized protocol to manage postoperative pain.
3. *Postoperative care*—early mobilization decreases risk of muscle loss and VTE, early feeding decreases nausea, vomiting, and decreases volume of intravenous (IV) fluids required. Effective analgesia decreases the dose of systemic opioids. Antiemetics for nausea/vomiting and laxatives to prevent constipation. Catheters, drains, vaginal packs, and IV drips should be removed as early as possible—to encourage mobilization and decreases secondary infection. After catheter removal, short-term voiding problems should be monitored with postvoid residual checks.

DISCHARGE

Once a patient has started mobilization, eating and drinking, passing flatus, and pain controlled by oral analgesia. Written information about emergency contact number, along with follow-up plans should be mentioned in discharge. Patient is also counseled about expected time of recovery and return to normal function.

SUGGESTED READING

1. Enhanced Recovery in Gynecology. The Obstetrician and Gynecologist. 2013;(15)4:263-8.

CHAPTER 59 Cerclage

■ CERVICAL INSUFFICIENCY

When uterine cervix is unable to retain a pregnancy in absence of uterine contractions, or labor, or both in second trimester leading to painless dilatation.

■ RISK FACTORS

Any surgical trauma to cervix due to conization, loop electrosurgical excision procedure (LEEP)/large loop excision of the transformation zone (LLETZ), mechanical cervical dilation during medical termination of pregnancy (MTP)/dilation and evacuation (D&E), or cervical injuries during delivery.

■ DIAGNOSIS

History of painless cervical dilation without any uterine contractions/labor leading to expulsion of pregnancy in second trimester, usually <24 weeks of pregnancy, **in absence of** bleeding, leaking, or an infection.

■ TREATMENT

Conservative treatment such as bed rest, limitation of activity, and vaginal pessary is not found to be effective. Surgical options include transvaginal/transabdominal cerclage.

■ CERCLAGE

Most common prophylactic intervention for pregnant women at risk of preterm birth/second trimester loss (stitch is inserted around cervix, to prevent recurrent loss). This not only provides support to "weak" cervix, but also maintains cervical length, and retains the endocervical mucus plug acting as an obstacle to ascending infection. Nomenclature based on indication is favored over previous terms (prophylactic/emergency/rescue/urgent).

History-indicated cerclage—as *prophylactic* at 11–14 weeks of pregnancy, in asymptomatic women with singleton pregnancy and ≥3 previous preterm birth *or* second trimester loss.

Ultrasound-indicated cerclage—as *therapeutic* at 14–24 weeks of pregnancy, in asymptomatic women with history of ≥1 spontaneous second trimester loss/preterm births, *and* short cervical length on transvaginal ultrasound (TVS). It is not recommended simply for funneling, i.e., dilatation of internal os on TVS in absence of cervical shortening ≤25 mm *or* in absence of O/H of preterm birth (PTB)/mid-trimester loss.

Ultrasound surveillance of cervical length advocated in women at high and intermediate risk:

- *High risk:* with previous PTB/second trimester loss (16–34 weeks), previous preterm prelabor rupture of membranes (PTPROM) <34 weeks, previous cerclage, known uterine variant, intrauterine adhesions, and history of trachelectomy.
- *At intermediate risk:* History of previous lower segment cesarean section (LSCS) at full dilatation, sig. cervical excisional surgery, i.e., LLETZ with excision depth >1 cm, >1 procedure, or cone biopsy.

Physical exam-indicated/emergency cerclage—as *salvage* in premature cervical dilatation with visible amniotic membrane in vagina diagnosed by per speculum (P/S) examination or ultrasonography (USG), in symptomatic women with vaginal discharge, bleeding or pressure symptoms, up to 27^{+6} weeks. It may delay birth by approximately 34 days in suitable cases, as compared to bed rest/expectant management alone. There is high chance of cerclage failure with advanced dilatation of cervix (>4 cm) or membrane prolapse beyond the external os.

■ CERCLAGE NOT RECOMMENDED

Multiple pregnancy, Mullerian anomalies, multiple D&E, or historyof cervical surgery such as cone biopsy, LEEP/LLETZ, or destructive procedures such as laser ablation or diathermy, if with no additional risk factors.

TYPES

- Transvaginal—McDonald—a purse-string suture placed at cervico-isthmus junction without mobilization of bladder/Shirodkar—purse-string suture placed after mobilization of bladder, to the level above cardinal ligaments.
- Transabdominal—via laparoscopy/laparotomy at cervico-isthmus junction, in previous unsuccessful transvaginal cerclage or extensive cervical surgery; performed preconceptually or in early pregnancy.
- Occlusion cerclage—External os is occluded by placement of a continuous nonabsorbable suture, causing retention of cervical mucus plug.

CONTRAINDICATIONS

Lethal fetal defect, intrauterine fetal demise, fetal distress, active preterm labor, bleeding, leaking (PPROM), or infection (chorioamnionitis).

COMPLICATIONS

Intraoperative injury to bladder, cervix, membrane rupture, bleeding, leaking, cervical injuries, if spontaneous labor occurs with suture in situ.

PREOPERATIVE MANAGEMENT

First trimester booking/viability scan + NT-NB scan to screen for aneuploidy before cerclage, singleton pregnancy, and rule out any lethal/major fetal anomaly. Anomaly scan before ultrasound-indicated or emergency cerclage. Maternal white blood cell (WBC) and C-reactive protein (CRP) for chorioamnionitis before insertion of emergency cerclage.

SUTURE REMOVAL

A transvaginal cervical cerclage should be removed before labor, usually between 36 and 37 weeks, unless planned for prelabor LSCS, in which suture removal could be delayed by this time. In established preterm labor, the cerclage should be removed to minimize injury to the cervix. A high (Shirodkar) cervical cerclage will require anesthesia for removal. In women with transabdominal cerclage requiring birth by CS, abdominal suture may be left in place.

In women with PPROM between 24 and 34 weeks and no evidence of infection/preterm labor, cerclage removal should be delayed for 48 hours, to facilitate in utero transfer. On other side, there is risk of neonatal and/or maternal sepsis if suture removal is delayed.

TREATMENT OF DELAYED MISCARRIAGE/ FETAL DEMISE WITH CERCLAGE

Complete evacuation through the stitch by suction-evacuation or by dilatation and evacuation (up to 18 weeks); or suture may be cut by posterior colpotomy failing which hysterotomy or LSCS may be done.

NOT RECOMMENDED

No role of routine amniocentesis before rescue/ultrasonography (USG) indicated cerclage, amnioreduction, no routine genital tract screening before cerclage, no routine perioperative tocolysis, no routine antibiotic prophylaxis, no bed rest, no abstinence from sexual intercourse, no routine progesterone (PGN) supplementation postcerclage, and no routine fetal fibronectin test.

SUGGESTED READING

1. ACOG practice bulletin number 142: Cerclage for the management of cervical insufficiency. Obstet Gynecol. 2014;123(2 Pt 1):372-9.
2. RCOG Green-top Guideline No.75. (2022). Cervical cerclage. [online] Available from https://www.rcog.org.uk/guidance/browse-all-guidance/green-top-guidelines/cervical-cerclage-green-top-guideline-no-75/ [Last accessed September, 2024].

CHAPTER 60

Pessaries

INTRODUCTION

Vaginal pessary is a device made of latex, silicone, or vinyl, which is inserted inside the vagina, in cases of uterovaginal prolapse, when patient is unfit/delays definitive surgery.

Action: When it is inserted inside the vagina, it stretches its walls and supporting connective tissues, in order to prevent the uterovaginal prolapse from sagging down.

INDICATIONS

- Patient unfit for surgery—due to old age, medical condition
- Not willing for surgery
- Wants pregnancy/during pregnancy
- To get time for healing of decubitus ulcer

TYPES

Support and space-occupying **(Figs. 1A to F)**:

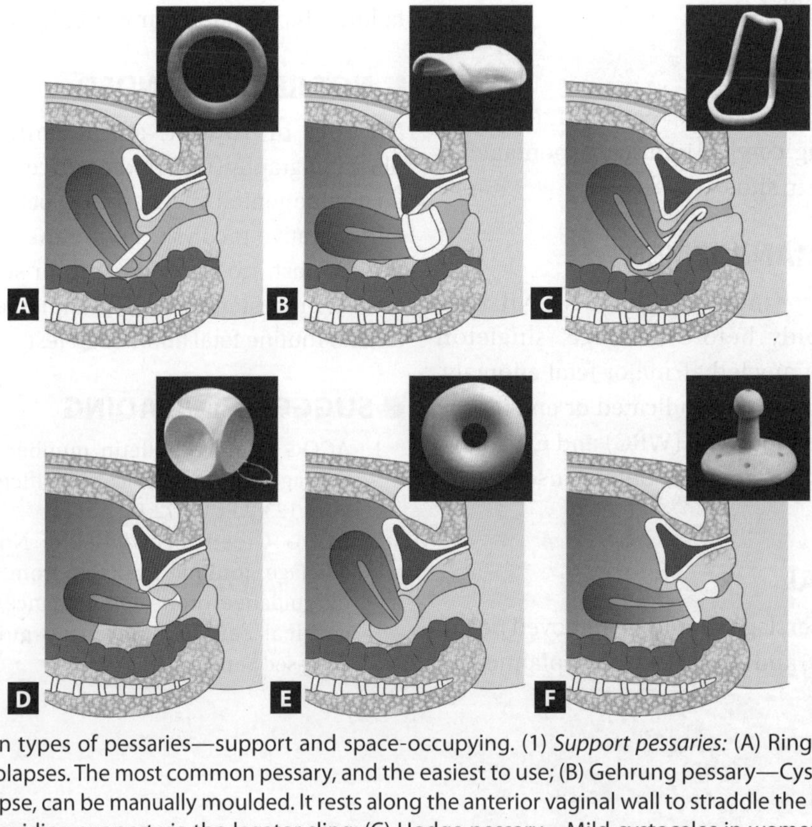

Figs. 1A to F: Two main types of pessaries—support and space-occupying. (1) *Support pessaries:* (A) Ring pessary—First and second degree uterovaginal prolapses. The most common pessary, and the easiest to use; (B) Gehrung pessary—Cystoceles and rectoceles, with or without uterine collapse, can be manually moulded. It rests along the anterior vaginal wall to straddle the bladder, and the lateral bars straddle the rectum, providing support via the legator sling; (C) Hodge pessary—Mild cystoceles in women with a narrow pubic arch, and for correcting a retroverted uterus. (2) *Space occupying pessaries:* (D) Cube pessary—Third degree uterovaginal prolapse. Maintains its position by creating suction between itself and the vaginal wall. Has no area for drainage and has to be removed nightly; (E) Donut pessary—Third degree uterovaginal prolapse. Remains in place by having a larger diameter than the genital hiatus. Usually latex, but an inflatable version allows for easy insertion and removal and an individualized fitting; (F) Gellhorn pessary—Third degree uterovaginal prolapse with decreased perineal support. Concave surface fits against the cervix or vaginal cuff. Stem should be positioned just behind the introitus, so perineum must be intact.

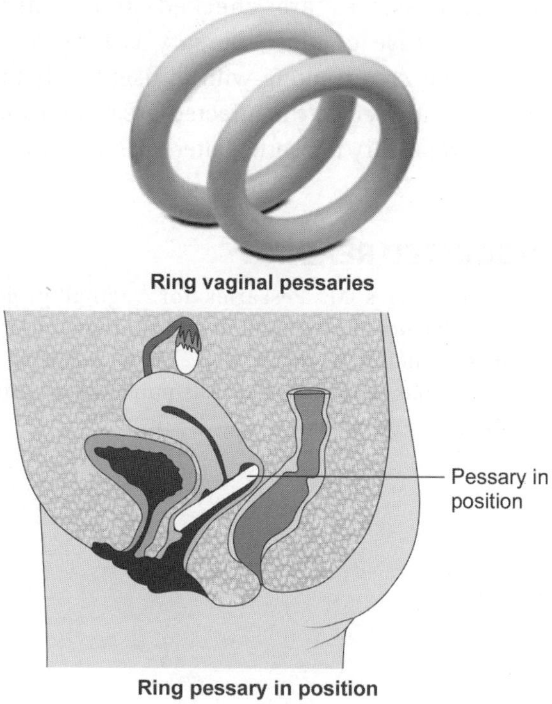

Fig. 2: Ring pessaries.

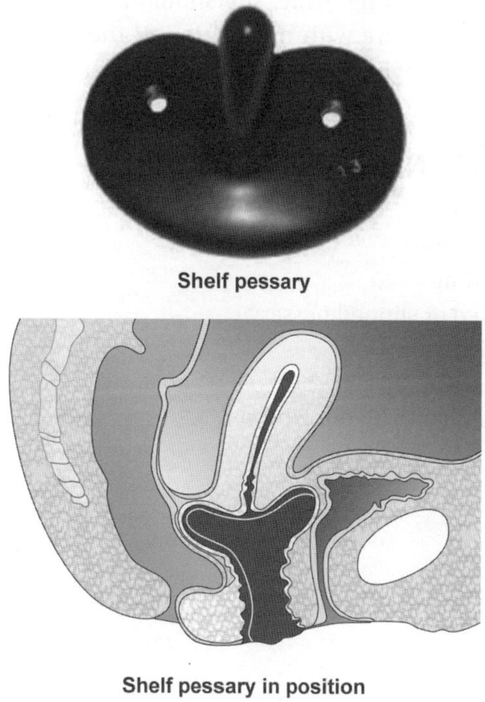

Fig. 3: Shelf pessaries.

- *Ring pessaries* **(Fig. 2)**—are one of the most commonly used support pessaries, which are soft and round, and do not interfere with sexual intercourse.
- *Shelf pessaries* **(Fig. 3)**—are one of the space-occupying pessaries, which are hard like a saucer with a knob, and interfere with sexual intercourse.
- *Gellhorn* **(Fig. 4)** pessaries are also type of space-occupying pessaries, similar to the shelf, but are soft with a knob, and interfere with sexual intercourse.

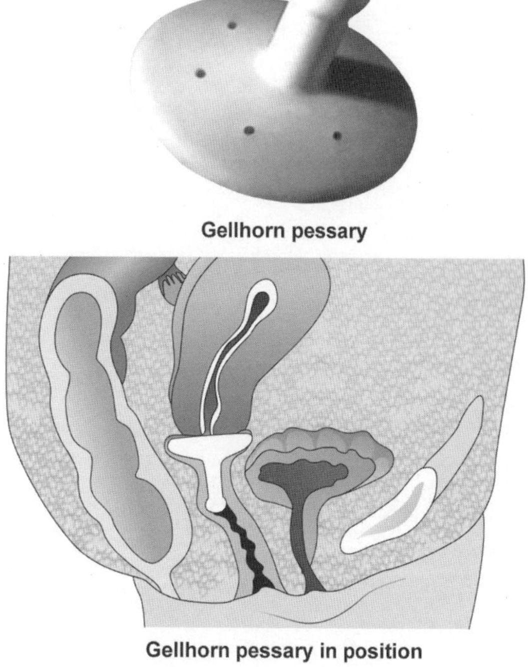

Fig. 4: Gellhorn pessaries.

METHOD OF INSERTION

All type of pessaries come in different sizes, and the correct size is determined by trial and error method while doing examination. Generally, ring pessaries are tried first but if the supporting pelvic floor muscles are not able to withstand pressure caused by it, then other types of pessaries are tested.

POSTPROCEDURE

The patient is advised to go to toilet and take a 15-20 minutes walk, to feel if the pessary is not tight enough causing discomfort or not loose enough to slip out.

Also, while passing urine, she should make sure that it does not interfere with micturition. If the pessary slips down or feels tight, it is replaced with smaller or larger size, respectively.

RISKS AND COMPLICATIONS

- Infection
- Ulceration
- Bleeding
- Moved or slipped pessary
- Difficult removal
- Pain
- Erosion into bladder/bowel

Hence, pessaries are checked and reinserted regularly. In case of ulcer, pessary is removed and local estrogen cream along with antiseptic (Betadine ointment) is advised to the affected area to encourage healing. New pessary reinserted after healing is complete (2–4 weeks).

SUGGESTED READING

1. Tam T, Davies M. Pessaries for vaginal prolapse: Critical factors to successful fit and continued use. OBG Management [Internet]. 2013;25(12):42-59. Available from: https://cdn.mdedge.com/files/s3fs-public/issues/articles/OBGM_1213_Tam.pdf.

CHAPTER 61

Diathermy/Electrosurgery in Gynecology

INTRODUCTION

Diathermy is use of *high frequency* electric current to produce heat in order to cut/coagulate tissue. Mains electricity is 50 Hz, while frequency in diathermy ranges from 300 KHz to 3 MHz, high frequency *avoids* muscle/nerve stimulation (spasm or twitching).

USES IN OBSTETRICS AND GYNECOLOGY

- Hemostasis in vaginal and abdominal surgery
- Incising deep layers of abdominal wall in laparotomy
- Laparoscopy—excision of endometrioma, ovarian drilling, cystectomy, myomectomy, hysterectomy, salpingectomy/salpingotomy/salpingo-oophorectomy.
- Colposcopy—large loop excision of the transformation zone (LLETZ)
- Hysteroscopy—endometrial resection/ablation, resection of endometrial polyps/submucosal fibroid.

TYPES OF CURRENT

- Cutting—continuous, low voltage
- Coagulate—interrupted, high voltage
- Blend—mixture of both cut and coagulation

TYPES OF DIATHERMY/ELECTROSURGERY (TABLE 1)

Monopolar

High frequency current passes from active electrode, through patient body to return electrode in diathermy plates (large surface area, placed on thigh, as close as possible to primary electrode), thus, patient is part of electric circuit. Active electrode is small so there is high current density and tissue heating; return electrode has large surface area to avoid heating effects as current density spreads over a large area and becomes less concentrated and low tissue heating. Advantages—easily available and

TABLE 1: Differences between monopolar and bipolar.

Monopolar devices	*Bipolar devices*
Lowest possible settings	Allow safety margin when close to vital structure, due to lateral thermal spread
Avoid patient end-plates on bony, scarred, hairy areas, and metal prosthesis	Avoid tension on tissue during activation, as this compromises coagulation
Vary surface area of active electrode to get desired effect without increasing power setting	Keep the jaws of instrument clean at all times (by wiping with wet swabs)
Short intermittent activation	Activate in short intermittent manner, and release tissue just before current flow terminated
Continuous low voltage waveform—cut mode for contact coagulation	If stuck to tissue, reapproximate jaws, and reactivate before releasing them
Avoid open activation	Avoid use in tissues with metal clips/staples-in situ
Avoid activation in close contact with another metal instrument	For good seal—avoid big tissue between jaws, and skeletonization of vessels before application
Use return electrode monitoring and active electrode monitoring technology	In comorbidities—liver disease, prolonged steroid use, diabetes, atherosclerosis, collagen disease, etc.—be extra cautious and use alternatives (∵ blood vessel affected)

easy to use, multiple modalities, used on small area/tissue for cutting (skin incision) and coagulation, can be attached to any instrument, and so no need to change. Disadvantages—can interfere with pacemaker and other electronic devices (insulin pump) function, arcing with metallic instruments, superficial burns if used for cutting with spirit-based skin preparation and pad not properly applied, ↑remote injuries, ↑temperature, and longer time to cool down.

Bipolar

Two active electrodes are combined in instruments, current passes between tips and not through the patient body, so there is no risk of wandering current and causing unintended damage/burns at distant sites. However, tissue between tips gets too hot so used for minimal required time. Advantages—safer than monopolar, less interference with pacemaker/other electronic devices function, less chance of remote injuries/burns, and preferred in endoscopic surgeries. Disadvantages—handle small amount of tissue, ↑chance of collateral damage, not suitable for cutting as power is low, arcing with metallic instruments, and heated tissue can damage bowel if in contact.

RISKS

- Toxic surgical smoke (fumes)
- Interfere with pacemaker/electronic device (insulin pump) function
- Arcing with metallic instruments and implants
- Superficial burns if used with alcohol/spirit-based skin preparation
- Burns under returning electrode if plate not properly applied
- Burns to viscus

PRECAUTIONS TO ENSURE SAFE DIATHERMY USE

- Proper training of staff/assistants using electrical energy.
- All equipment to be regularly checked and serviced [World Health Organization (WHO) surgical safety check].
- Proper suction of surgical smoke (fumes) during surgery.
- Suction-irrigation regularly to cool down instruments and diathermized area.
- Bipolar should be preferred whenever possible.
- No uninsulated metal come in contact with patient (provide alternative electrical path).
- Split plate return electrode checked for proper application over large well-vascularized muscle mass [avoid over scar or keloid (less vascularized)/irregular body contours or bony areas].
- If unilateral artificial hip → place return electrode on opposite side, if bilateral artificial hips → place on back, if pacemaker, avoid using monopolar.
- During laparoscopy, instruments to be kept in vision always and make sure bowel away.
- Place all electrodes in insulated sheath when not in use, and do not leave it on patient's abdomen or held in assistant's/nurse's hand.
- Use well-insulated electrodes and check to rule out insulation failure (invisible bowel injury).
- Activate the electrodes only when whole area transmitting current is under vision, to avoid direct coupling with other conducting instruments → injury outside view.
- All metal/all plastic trocars should be used to avoid capacitative coupling.
- Always use isolated electrosurgical generator, brief intermittent activation (avoid prolonged activation).
- Use low voltage waveforms/low power where possible.

DIRECT COUPLING

In laparoscopy, when an active electrode touches another metal instrument or conductor, resulting in electrical burn, tissue damage and increased risk of infection to the tissue/organs in contact.

Prevention of direct coupling:
- Always visualize the electrode and ensure the uninsulated section of the active electrode is visible before activating it
- Avoid touching any other conductive instruments before activating the electrode
- Use a low power current
- Use an active electrode monitoring system (AEM)—a system to monitor the active electrode
- Use disposable instruments as they are less likely to have insulation failure than reusable instruments.

CAPACITATIVE COUPLING

Transfer of electric current through intact insulation, from an active electrode into adjacent conducting material without direct contact. Monopolar lap instruments create large capacitator, energy transferred through capacitative coupling depends on capacitor size, activation mode, and voltage output, e.g., when active electrode passed down a metal suction irrigator/hybrid cannula (metal cannula with plastic gripper), insulated shaft of active electrode touches nontargeted tissue, e.g., bowel/adhesion, active electrode induces current in nearby cold instrument or into adjacent tissue; most common with single port laparoscopy.

Prevention of capacitative coupling:

- Avoid hybrid cannula
- Lower electrosurgical unit power settings
- Using "cut" rather coagulation mode
- Use short interrupted activation
- Avoid open activation
- Not operate close to metal in operative field
- Use of adaptive electrosurgical technology which measures tissues impedance during activation and modify output voltage accordingly—tissue response generators
- Use of active electrode monitoring—most effective way of dealing with strong current caused by insulation failure and capacitative coupling.

MANAGEMENT OF DIATHERMY BURN

Depends on site/size/degree:

- At skin site (return electrode) → remove machine immediately and report to biomedical team, communicate with anesthetist/surgical team/tissue-viability nurse → examine whole patient and assess degree of burns for tissue viability → ensure adequate analgesia, antibiotics, and local cream → possibly plastic surgery and grafting.
- Internal organs—bowel resection and anastomosis, bladder and urethral injury repair, and vascular repair.

SUGGESTED READING

1. El-Sayed M, Mohamed S, Saridogan E. Safe use of electrosurgery in gynaecological laparoscopic surgery. The Obstetrician & Gynaecologist. 2019;22(1):9-20.

CHAPTER 62

Endometrial Ablation

HEAVY MENSTRUAL BLEEDING DEFINITION

Excessive menstrual blood loss, which interferes with a woman's physical, social, emotional, and/or material quality of life occurring alone or in combination with other symptoms. Management options are medical [Tranexamic acid/Mefenamic acid; hormonal—Levonorgestrel-releasing intrauterine system (LNG-IUS), combined oral contraceptive (COC)] and surgical—endometrial ablation and hysterectomy.

ENDOMETRIAL ABLATION

Technique that aims to permanently destroy the functionally active endometrial glands, which are located in the endomyometrial junction and up to 5 mm of the myometrium to reduce heavy menstrual bleeding (HMB). A minimally invasive alternative to hysterectomy, also avoids chronic use of medications and offered to women who have completed their family/no desire for future fertility with uterus no larger than 10 weeks of pregnancy [National Institute for Health and Care Excellence (NICE)].

CONTRAINDICATIONS

Endometrial hyperplasia, endometrial cancer, desirous for pregnancy, active pelvic inflammatory disease (PID), currently using intrauterine device (IUD), uterine anomaly (septum/unicornuate), myometrial thinning following uterine surgery [C-section (CS), myomectomy], post-menopausal bleeding, Lynch syndrome, on Tamoxifen, risk factors for endometrial cancer (Ca)—hypertension (HTN), obesity, diabetes mellitus (DM), and chronic anovulation.

FACTORS ASSOCIATED WITH TREATMENT FAILURE

Large uterine cavity size >10 weeks, adenomyosis, intra-cavity lesions—fibroids and polyps, multiparity (>5), young age, acute—ante/retroflexion, or ante/retroversion.

FIRST-GENERATION TECHNIQUES

Refers to **hysteroscopic** procedures, performed under direct vision and require distension of uterine cavity using a nonionic fluid medium (glycine).

- *Transcervical resection of endometrium (TCRE)*—involves resecting the endometrium using a 3 mm electrosurgical loop with an operative hysteroscope, i.e., resectoscope. Glycine used with monopolar current (blend at 80–100 W) and normal saline used with bipolar (Versapoint) current thus avoiding risk of glycine overload causing ammonia toxicity [~transurethral resection syndrome (TUR) syndrome by urologists]. Disadvantage with normal saline (NS) is as blood is miscible, it compromises the surgical field in heavy bleeding. It has the longest learning curve, and the highest risk of complications.
- *Roller ball endometrial ablation*—uses a roller ball electrode instead of a loop through the resectoscope to ablate the endometrial cavity, but without removal of tissue. It is safer over areas where myometrium is relatively thin, e.g., cornual region or over a CS scar as moving faster over thinned areas leads to less depth of penetration or can be avoided altogether. Less complications as compared to TCRE.
- *Endometrial laser ablation*—after distending the uterine cavity with NS, a 600-µm flexible quartz optical fiber is inserted through operating channel of the hysteroscope that transmits neodymium-doped yttrium aluminum garnet (Nd:YAG) laser energy (50–80 W) to the endometrium and drawn over endometrial surface to achieve destruction up to superficial myomerium. Rarely used now in view of costs, prolonged operating times and safety issues.

SECOND-GENERATION TECHNIQUES

Not performed under direct vision, except for hydrothermal ablation, thus less dependent on surgeon's skills, and quicker to learn and safer to use.

TABLE 1: Types of thermal balloons.

Systems	Fluid used	Temperature	Pressure (mm Hg)
Thermachoice III	5% Dextrose	87°C	160–180
Cavaterm	5% Dextrose	78°C	230–240
Thermablate	Glycerine	173°C	220
Menotreat	Normal saline	85°C	200

- *Thermal balloon ablation* (**Table 1**)—consists of a catheter and a silicone balloon filled with circulating hot liquid at high pressures to ablate the endometrial cavity, e.g., Thermachoice III Uterine Balloon Therapy Cavaterm, Thermablate Endometrial Ablation System, and Menotreat balloon.

  Treatment time for all these devices varies between 2 and 10 minutes. Combination of high temperature and high pressure causes endovascular coagulation in the endometrial lining, resulting in an immediate blistery, blanched effect followed by fibrosis causing permanent inactive endometrium. Contraindications (CI)—classical cesarean section or history of transmural myomectomy. Endometrial preparation not required as endometrium is compressed by balloon pressure.
- *Microwave endometrial ablation*—metal tube with dielectric filling and radiating tip that propagates microwave energy at 9.2 GHz into uterine cavity, treatment time <3 minutes. Electromagnetic waves generated in magnetron produces a hemispherical arc of heat 70–80°C at tip, which is drawn over inside uterine cavity. There is continuous temperature display and the device shuts off power at 90°C.
- *Novasure endometrial ablation*—an expanding bipolar electrode array with porous fabric mesh inserted into uterine cavity and suction is continuously applied to bring the endometrium into its contact, thus removing hot gas, blood, and debris from uterine cavity. Power is delivered from control unit according to uterine cavity (maximum 180 W) and shuts off automatically at 2 minutes (average treatment time—90 seconds).
- *Hydrothermal ablation*—performed under direct hysteroscopic vision and endometrial destruction is achieved by free circulating heated saline at 90°C in the cavity under pressure of 50–55 mm Hg, to prevent leakage from tubes/cervix during 10 minutes treatment. A tight seal at the cervix is essential to prevent leakage of hot saline and avoid vaginal burns. Not effective with cavity length <6 cm/>10.5 cm, with intramural fibroids >4 cm or with intracavity fibroids. Advantage is as performed under direct vision, irregular cavities or with fibroids can be treated. But there is need to induce endometrial thinning with gonadotropin-releasing hormone (GnRH) analogs prior to treatment.
- *Her option*—uses gas mixture as coolant, which is circulated by a control unit in a closed system. Passage of gas through a small diameter orifice at tip of probe causes rapid expansion and drop in temperature of coolant to –115°C to –125°C, at pressure of 300–350 psi, forming a cryozone done under ultrasonography (USG) treatment time longer 12–15 minutes.

Preoperative preparation—preoperative evaluation, risk assessment, endometrial sampling, assessment of uterine cavity, rule out pregnancy, treat genital tract infection, and informed consent—benefits (↓volume of uterine bleeding, but neither produce amenorrhea nor regularize irregular periods), risks, and alternatives. With first-generation techniques, endometrial preparation with GnRH analogs reduces operating times and fluid absorption but increases cervical resistance, thus making dilatation difficult. Pretreatment do not offer any advantage with second-generation techniques and is associated with a higher incidence of adverse effects.

COMPLICATIONS

Uterine perforation, hemorrhage, hematometra (due to intrauterine scarring), and infection—endometritis, myometritis, PID, and pelvic abscess; apart from method-related like fluid overload with first-generation techniques or vaginal burns with hot water ablation.

SUGGESTED READING

1. Parkin DE. Endometrial ablation techniques. The Obstetrician & Gynaecologist. 2011;2(1):35-8.
2. Progress in gynecology.
3. Recent advances in gynecology.

CHAPTER 63

Uterine Artery Embolization

DEFINITION

Uterine artery embolization (UAE) is a minimally invasive treatment for abnormal uterine bleeding (AUB), a percutaneous angiographic procedure performed with video fluoroscopic imaging.

INDICATIONS

- Symptomatic fibroids
- Atonic postpartum hemorrhage (PPH)
- Bleeding after C-section (CS)
- Bleeding after gynecological surgery
- Arteriovenous malformation
- Gestational trophoblastic diseases

Indications for fibroid embolization include the following:

- Symptomatic fibroids
- Medical condition contraindicating surgery, i.e., unfit for surgery
- Not willing for surgery or unwilling to receive BT during surgery
- Not responded to conservative treatment or surgery
- Fibroid with infertility—(relative) if myomectomy is contraindicated/refused

CONTRAINDICATIONS

- *Absolute:*
  - Asymptomatic fibroid
  - Current genital tract infection [pelvic inflammatory disease (PID)]
  - Doubtful diagnosis, i.e., uterine malignancy
  - Pregnancy
  - Unwilling for hysterectomy (social/cultural reasons), if required due to complications
- *Relative contraindications (CI):*
  - Narrow-stalked pedunculated submucosal fibroids (may need hysteroscopic removal)
  - Large intracavity submucosal fibroids (may cause cervical obstruction, sepsis)
  - Pedunculated subserosal fibroids (may need laparoscopic removal)
  - Large fibroids mainly associated with bulk symptoms (pressure symptoms, frequency, urgency, and urinary incontinence—as volume reduction may not be sufficient)
  - Desire to preserve fertility

FIBROID WITH INFERTILITY

Intracavity and intramural fibroids act by mechanical distortion, but even if cavity is normal it may interfere with fertility by effects on uterine blood flow, impaired embryo implantation, or abnormal sperm migration. During pregnancy it may lead to miscarriages, red degeneration causing pain, preterm labor, mechanical complications in labor, and postpartum hemorrhage (PPH). Hence, women who desire fertility but experience infertility or recurrent miscarriage due to fibroids (multiple) may be offered UAE, whereas for single large fibroid myomectomy is better. Besides, UAE may interfere with placental blood flow and increases chance of uterine rupture due to myometrial ischemia, however, myomectomy causes uterine scarring, adhesion formation, focal myometrial weakness, and uterine perforation.

Pretreatment evaluation—Multidisciplinary team (MDT) involving gynecologist, interventional radiologist, and specialist nurse. Counseling and consent regarding procedure and outcome, duration of hospital stay, recovery time, complications—short-term/medium term (up to 5 years) and long-term—may require further treatment. Preoperative gonadotropin-releasing hormone (GnRH) agonists to decrease fibroid volume, magnetic resonance imaging (MRI) for fibroid mapping, rule out pregnancy by urine pregnancy test (UPT), treat any genital tract infection, prophylactic antibiotics, and thromboprophylaxis.

Procedure—an up-to-date dedicated fixed C-arm fluoroscopic unit supporting "road mapping" and dose reduction modes (pulsed fluoroscopy) with trained radiographer to minimize radiation. In parenteral conscious sedation and analgesia, right-sided (or bilateral) percutaneous femoral arterial access done and catheter is manipulated under fluoroscopic guidance to uterine artery via anterior division of internal iliac artery. Embolic agents like polyvinyl alcohol (diameter 300–750 micrometers) injected under fluoroscopic control till complete stasis in uterine artery, avoiding reflux, and nontarget embolization. Continuous monitoring of vitals with resuscitation facilities should be available. After completion of procedure, catheter is removed and hemostasis checked, total procedure timing 30–90 minutes.

Complications-immediate (periprocedural)—local, e.g., groin hematoma, arterial thrombosis, dissection, and pseudoaneurysm, arterial puncture, and spasm of uterine artery; reaction to iodinated contrast media, necrosis of gluteus maximus muscle or limbs, nontarget embolization of ovarian artery leading to permanent amenorrhea. Early (<30 days)—postembolization syndrome [pain, nausea, fever, malaise associated with raised inflammatory markers and white blood cell (WBC) count—symptomatically managed]; urinary tract infection (UTI) and deep vein thrombosis (DVT) (rare).

Late (>30 days)—vaginal discharge (may become infective), fibroid expulsion and impaction, endometritis leading to abscess, pelvic peritonitis, septicemia and multiple organ dysfunction syndrome (MODS) may require emergency hysterectomy. Besides, amenorrhea due to ovarian insufficiency and sexual dysfunction due to disturbed blood supply may also occur.

Follow-up—urgently in case of complications, otherwise routine follow-up after 6 months postprocedure. Thorough clinical assessment with imaging is mandatory.

Outcome—most patients (~80%) report improvement of abnormal uterine bleeding up to 5–10 years after UAE, however one-third may require hysterectomy within 5 years of it.

SUGGESTED READING

1. Davies R, Parker M, Basu A, Alleemudder D. The clinical applications of interventional radiological techniques in obstetrics and gynecology. The Obstetrician & Gynecologist. 2023;(25)2:131-9.

CHAPTER 64

Urinary Tract Injuries During Gynecological Surgeries

INTRODUCTION

Most common type of major visceral complication during pelvic surgeries. They are of two types—bladder injuries and ureteric injuries.

BLADDER INJURIES

Common site of bladder injury is in midline, above interureteric bar, because these occur during bladder dissection from cervix during hysterectomy. Key factors are—surgical experience, complexity of operation, and distorted/normal anatomy. Risk factors for distorted pelvic anatomy are—endometriosis, adhesions, cancer, severe urogenital prolapse, obesity, and pregnancy.

Prevention

Knowledge of anatomy, meticulous dissection technique, and understanding of electrosurgery are prerequisites for safe surgery. To prevent electro-surgical complications—inspect insulation of all instruments before use, power should be used at lowest possible setting, active electrode monitoring (AEM) should be done by using tissue response generators, monopolar diathermy (cut) should be used at low voltage, bipolar should always be preferred over monopolar because patient's body does not form part of circuit, short intermittent activation done while using, not to use if in direct contact/nearby other instrument, and ensure that during activation both tips of bipolar forceps is in direct view.

Recognition (Intraoperative)

About half of all bladder injuries are not recognized during primary surgery. It can be obvious directly via obvious cystotomy and/or urinary leakage; indirectly by noting hematuria in catheter and Urobag. Confirmed by cystoscopy and/or instillation of Methylene blue (200–300 mL) colored saline through urethra into bladder exhibits site and size of injury, intraoperatively.

Recognition (Postoperative)

Hematuria, delayed recovery, suprapubic pain, and oliguria due to urinary leakage per vagina. Chemical peritonitis due to peritoneal irritation by urine leads to diffuse lower abdominal pain, distension, and ileus. These appear within first 48 hours of operation and characterized by absence of tenderness. Thermal injuries usually manifest after 10–14 days of operation, characterized by urinary leak per vaginum [vesicovaginal fistula (VVF)]/ into peritoneal cavity.

Investigation

Computed tomography (CT)-urogram, retrograde cystography, and cystoscopy help to confirm the site and size of injuries. In VVF—three swab test and magnetic resonance imaging (MRI) can be diagnostic.

Management

Multidisciplinary team (MDT) involving urologist and/ or urogynecologist. Injury repaired in two layers using a 2-0/3-0 absorbable suture like polyglactin, in running nonlocking fashion (0.5–1 cm apart, starting 0.5–1 cm lateral to cystotomy angles). For small defect, "figure of 8" suture may be enough. Injuries involving trigone need ureteral stenting and thus patency of both ureters and urethra should be confirmed before repair. Thermal injury may require debridement before repair. Ideally, repair should be checked intraoperatively for water tightness by methylene blue instilled through catheter, and catheter kept for 2 weeks along with antibiotics. Prior to catheter removal, repair confirmed by retrograde cystography.

URETERIC INJURIES

Incidence higher with laparoscopic > abdominal > vaginal hysterectomies. Most common site is at infundibulopelvic ligament, at uterine clamp or at vaginal angles.

Prevention

Knowledge of anatomy, meticulous dissection technique, and understanding of electrosurgery are prerequisites as for bladder injury prevention. In complex cases like endometriosis, preoperative intravenous urography (IVU)/ MRI/stenting may be an option. Intraoperative identifying ureteric peristalsis is helpful. It is important to dissect, expose, and mobilize the ureter in pelvic endometriosis, pelvic adhesions, cervical fibroids, big ovarian cysts, etc., by medial-to-lateral blunt sweeping technique so that it will carry its blood vessels in its adventitia (mobilized up to 15 cm provided its vascular supply is preserved). Electrosurgery used with caution in its proximity. Finally, adequate dissection of bladder from cervix carries ureters out of the field, decreases the risk of injury.

Recognition (Intraoperative)

Only one-third cases are recognized intraoperative. Intravenous (IV) Indigo carmine given intraoperatively will color urine blue in 5–10 minutes, thus identifying site of leak. Cystoscopy visualizes ureteric orifices and also urinary jet, with presence of blood. Ureteroscopy, intraoperative stenting without resistance (therapeutic also), antegrade/retrograde IV ureteropyelography are also helpful in making the diagnosis.

Seven types of ureteric injury are—angulation, crush, ligation, thermal, laceration, transection, and resection.

Recognition (Postoperative)

If patient fails to recover after major pelvic surgery along with flank pain and flank tenderness, hematuria, oliguria, or watery vaginal loss present within the first 48 hours of an acute injury. Uroperitoneum/urinoma may lead to abscess formation, sepsis, and electrolyte imbalance. Thermal injury leads to delayed necrosis and presents with fistula 10–14 days postoperatively. Ultrasonography (USG), computed tomography (CT) urogram, and cysto-ureteroscopy help to identify the site of injury.

Management

Principles—preferably by laparoscopy—careful dissection to avoid devascularization, careful debridement to avoid shortening for reanastomosis; suturing should be water-tight, tension-free, in spatulated or fish-mouth pattern, with delayed absorbable sutures; proper and continuous urine drainage via ureteric stenting, Foley's catheter, ± retroperitoneal drain; and to increase vascularity cover the site by omental flap.

Minor crush/needle injuries—conservative treatment, if ureter is viable and integrity is maintained, i.e., peristalsis and perfusion maintained with no urine leak.

Obstruction, crush, small thermal, and ligature injuries—ureteral stenting, to prevent stenosis and helps in healing, but if more extensive deep thermal injury, excision of affected part and ureteral reanastomosis/ reimplantation needed.

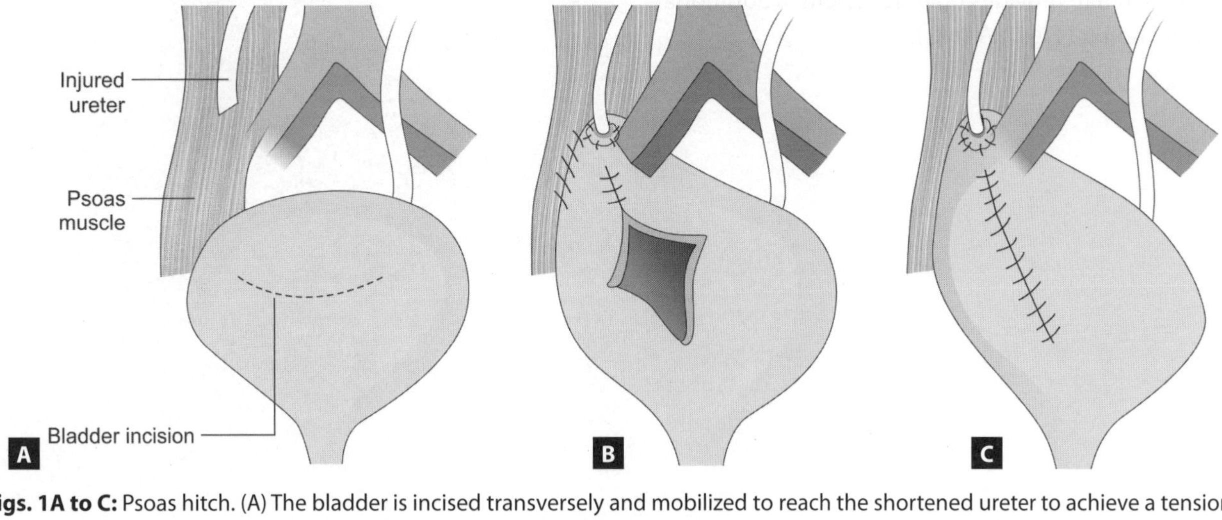

Figs. 1A to C: Psoas hitch. (A) The bladder is incised transversely and mobilized to reach the shortened ureter to achieve a tension-free anastomosis; (B) The bladder is fixed to the psoas muscle; (C) The incision repaired in a vertical manner which allows "elongation" of the bladder.

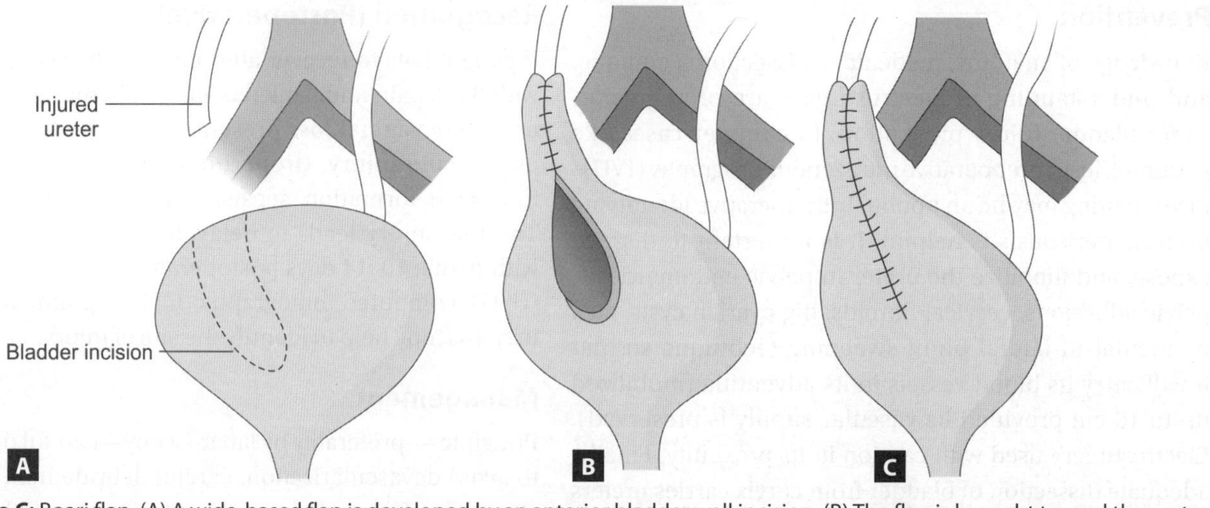

Figs. 2A to C: Boari flap. (A) A wide-based flap is developed by an anterior bladder wall incision; (B) The flap is brought toward the ureter to achieve a tension-free anastomosis; (C) The bladder incision is closed in a tubular manner to allow up to 12–15 cm of additional length.

Ureteric lacerations—suturing and stenting.

Transection/resection, treatment is site-specific. Upper one-third of the ureter → end-to-end reanastomosis, i.e., ureteroureterostomy. In middle one-third → uretero-ureterostomy or transureteroureterostomy, i.e., end-to-side anastomosis of injured ureter with the contralateral healthy ureter. Lower one-third → ureteroneocystostomy, i.e., ureter is reimplanted into bladder. To decrease tension at site of anastomosis, a psoas hitch (bladder fixed to iliopsoas muscle) **(Figs. 1A to C)** or a Boari flap (dome of bladder is cut, an oblique flap created, and closed vertically) Boari flap provides up to 12–15 cm of additional length to the ureter **(Figs. 2A to C)**.

SUGGESTED READING

1. Jeffery S. Procedures in obstetrics and gynaecology [Internet]. 2010 https://www.glowm.com/pdf/Textbook-UniversityOfCapeTown-Procedures%20in%20OBGYN-CC%20BY%20NC%20SA.pdf.
2. Jha S, Coomarasamy A, Chan KK. Ureteric injury in obstetric and gynaecological surgery. Obstet Gynaecol [Internet]. 2004;6(4):203-8.
3. Minas V, Gul N, Aust T, Doyle M, Rowlands D. Urinary tract injuries in laparoscopic gynaecological surgery; prevention, recognition and management. Obstet Gynaecol [Internet]. 2014;16(1):19-28.

CHAPTER 65 Manual Vacuum Aspiration

DEFINITION

Procedure that uses a vacuum source to remove an embryo or fetus through the cervix, up to gestational age of 10 weeks.

SELECTION CRITERIA

- Motivational multiparas
- Hemodynamically stable
- Crown-rump length (CRL) <25 mm
- No infection
- Nulliparous, if well motivated

INDICATIONS

- Early pregnancy termination
- Incomplete miscarriage
- Endometrial biopsy
- Menstrual regulation

CONTRAINDICATIONS

- Pregnancy >10 weeks
- Retained products of conception (RPOC) >5 cm
- Postpartum RPOC
- Associated with infection
- Anatomical—cervical stenosis, uterine malformations
- Female factors—panic attacks, hemorrhagic disorders, and allergy to local anesthetics (LA)

PREREQUISITES

- Written and informed consent
- Empty bladder
- Cervical preparation with prostaglandin E1 (PGE1) 2–3 hours before
- Pain relief—nonsteroidal anti-inflammatory drugs (NSAIDs) [Paracetamol (PCM) if asthmatic/renal dis]
- Resuscitation trolley
- Charging syringe
- Correct size Karman's cannula

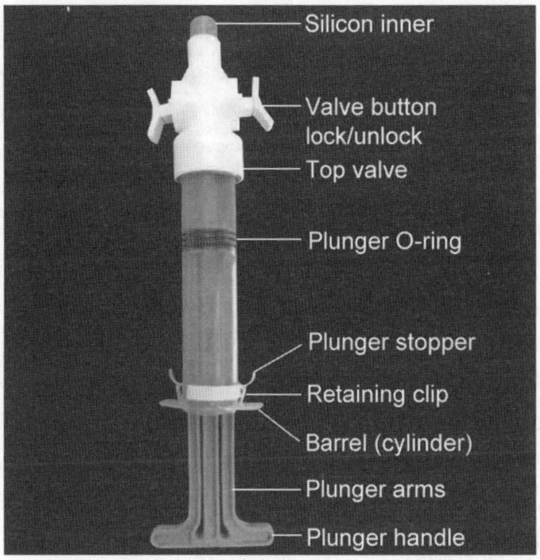

Fig. 1: Parts of MVA syringe. (MVA: manual vacuum aspiration)

Parts of instrument **(Fig. 1)**—Cannula, valve liner, valve, barrel, and plunger with O-ring.

Adaptors of appropriate sizes (according to cannulas) (4 mm—yellow, 5 mm—light green, 6 mm—blue, 7 mm—brown, 8 mm—white, 9 mm—tan, 10 mm—dark green, 11 mm—dark blue, 12 mm—needs no adapter).

PROCEDURE (FIG. 2)

- *Step I:* Patient preparation—analgesics, prophylactic antibiotics, empty bladder, per speculum, and bimanual pelvic examination to rule out infection, bleeding, and incomplete abortion.
- *Step II:* Antiseptic preparation of cervix—antiseptic soaked sponge to clean external os, start at os and spiral outward without retracing areas, repeat until os has been completely covered by antiseptics.
- *Step III:* Paracervical block—20 cc of 1% Lignocaine; inject a small amount (1–2 cc) into cervix at tenaculum site (12 o'clock). Inject remaining Lignocaine in equal amount (3–4 cc) at cervicovaginal junction at 2, 4, 8, and 10 o'clock position. Always aspirate before injecting to prevent intravascular injection of Lignocaine.

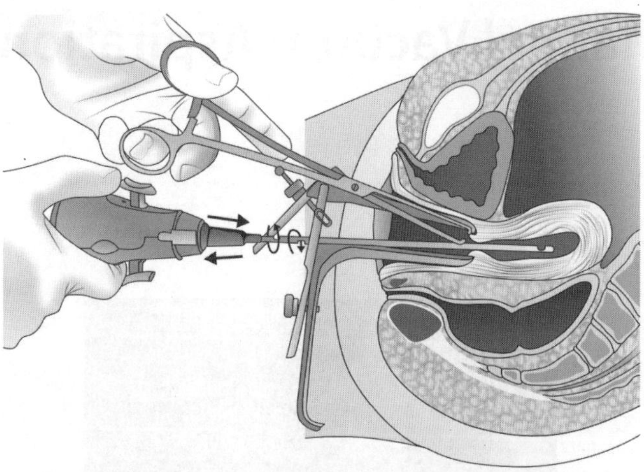

Fig. 2: MVA in action. (MVA: manual vacuum aspiration)

- *Step IV:* Dilate cervix—"No touch" technique when dilating the cervix and during aspiration, i.e., instruments that enter the uterine cavity should not touch gloved hands, patient's skin, vaginal walls, or unsterile parts of instrument tray before entering cervix. Use mechanical dilators/progressive larger cannulas to gently dilate cervix to right uterine size.
- *Step V:* Insert cannula—while applying traction to tenaculum, insert cannula through the cervix, just past the internal os, into uterine cavity. Do not insert forcefully.
- *Step VI:* Prepare aspirator—position the plunger all the way inside the cylinder → put collar stop in place with tabs in cylinder holes → push valve buttons down and forward until they lock → pull plunger back until arms snap outward and catch on cylinder base.
- *Step VII:* Suction uterine contents—attach the prepared aspirator to cannula (already inserted inside uterus) → release vacuum by pressing both valve buttons → evacuate the contents of uterus by gentle slow rotation of cannula 180° in each direction, using an in-and-out motion. When procedure is finished, depress the buttons, and disconnect cannula from the aspirator (or withdraw cannula and aspirator).
- *Step VIII:* Inspect tissue—empty contents of aspirator into a container, strain material, float in water/vinegar, and view with light from beneath. Inspect tissue for products of conception (POC), complete evacuation, or molar tissue. If inspection is inconclusive, reaspiration or other evaluation may be necessary.
- *Step IX:* Perform any concurrent procedures—when procedure is complete, proceed with contraception/others, e.g., intrauterine contraceptive device (IUCD) insertion/cervical tear repair.
- *Step X:* Immediately postprocedure—reassure the patient that procedure is finished, ensure she is escorted to recovery area. Immediately process/discard all instruments, according to local policy guidelines.

Signs of uterine cavity being empty:

- Red/pink foam without tissue seen passing through cannula
- Gritty sensation felt as cannula passes over surface of evacuated uterus
- Uterus contracts/grips the cannula
- Patient complaining of cramps/pain indicating uterus is contracting.

COMPLICATIONS

Injury to cervix/uterus (during cannula insertion), bleeding, infection, incomplete evacuation, anaphylaxis due to inadvertent, intravenous (IV) injection of Lignocaine.

SUGGESTED READING

1. Allie S. Evacuation of the uterus. In: Jeffery S (Ed). Procedures in obstetrics and gynaecology [Internet]. 2010. [cited 2024 Oct 9]. Available from: https://www.glowm.com/pdf/Textbook-UniversityOfCapeTown-Procedures%20in%20OBGYN-CC%20BY%20NC%20SA.pdf.

NOTES

NOTES

Index

Page numbers followed by *b* refer to box, *f* refer to figure, *fc* refer to flowchart, and *t* refer to table.

A

B

C

D

L

M

Q

R

S

T

U

V

W

Z